Botulinum Toxin in Urology

Michael B. Chancellor • Christopher P. Smith

Botulinum Toxin in Urology

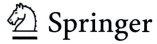

Authors
Dr. Michael B. Chancellor
Department of Urology
Oakland University,
Willam Beaumont School of Medicine
Royal Oak, MI 48073
USA
chancellormb@gmail.com

Dr. Christopher P. Smith
The Scott Department of Urology
Baylor College of Medicine
Houston, TX 77030
USA
cps@bcm.edu

ISBN 978-3-642-03579-1   e-ISBN 978-3-642-03580-7
DOI 10.1007/978-3-642-03580-7
Springer Heidelberg Dordrecht London New York

Library of Congress Control Number: 2011928409

© Springer-Verlag Berlin Heidelberg 2011
This work is subject to copyright. All rights are reserved, whether the whole or part of the material is concerned, specifically the rights of translation, reprinting, reuse of illustrations, recitation, broadcasting, reproduction on microfilm or in any other way, and storage in data banks. Duplication of this publication or parts thereof is permitted only under the provisions of the German Copyright Law of September 9, 1965, in its current version, and permission for use must always be obtained from Springer. Violations are liable to prosecution under the German Copyright Law.

The use of general descriptive names, registered names, trademarks, etc. in this publication does not imply, even in the absence of a specific statement, that such names are exempt from the relevant protective laws and regulations and therefore free for general use.

Product liability: The publishers cannot guarantee the accuracy of any information about dosage and application contained in this book. In every individual case the user must check such information by consulting the relevant literature.

Cover design: eStudioCalamar, Figueres/Berlin

Printed on acid-free paper

Springer is part of Springer Science+Business Media (www.springer.com)

Foreword

Europe, North America and Asia

Professor Christopher Chapple

Dear Colleagues,

I would like to congratulate Michael Chancellor and Christopher Smith on this very interesting overview of the use of botulinum toxin in the treatment of urological disorders.

It is now clearly recognised that as a biological agent, the various formulations of botulinum toxin differ markedly in terms of their content, potency and potential site of action. There is no adequately controlled comparative data currently available contrasting one formulation of botulinum toxin with another. Most of the evidence base relating to the utilisation of botulinum toxin is from studies using onabotulinumtoxinA.

We have phase II dose ranging data for onabotulinumtoxinA in idiopathic detrusor overactivity and phase III data with its use in the treatment of neurogenic detrusor overactivity in both multiple sclerosis patients and spinal cord injury patients recently reported at international meetings.

This excellent overview comprehensively covers safety and general principles, aetiology and aspects of potential mechanisms of action and looks at the use of treatment for bladder, prostate and pelvic floor disorders. In addition there are interesting sections on the role of botulinum toxin in medicine, with a consideration of health economics.

Currently botulinum toxin proves to be enormously useful in the management of both idiopathic and neurogenic detrusor overactivity in our practice and we eagerly await the results of the phase III dataset with onabotulinumtoxinA.

Although we have limited evidence base as to the volume of injection to be used and the site of injection, it is our practice to use 0.5 ml injection, each containing 10 units of onabotulinumtoxinA and our standard therapy has been using 200 units, but in view of the recently reported dose ranging study with onabotulinumtoxinA in idiopathic detrusor overactivity, we are considering utilising 100 units as primary treatment of these patients and then up-titrating as necessary.

All of our patients at present are informed that the treatment is currently off-label and warned about the potential consequences of this therapy, in particular relating to urinary retention, which seems to be the main potential side effect; symptoms of cystitis do occur but we routinely use antibiotic prophylaxis. We tend to inject onabotulinumtoxinA across the base of the bladder.

OnabotulinumtoxinA in our practice has been used for sensory bladder disorder with interesting early results when injected into the trigone. We have not utilised it for the management of benign prostatic obstruction or sphincteric or pelvic floor disorders.

In my view it has proved to be a very useful treatment for both idiopathic and neurogenic detrusor overactivity. The use of onabotulinumtoxinA still has to be adequately investigated in painful bladder syndrome, where there is very limited evidence base, and to date its use in other conditions, in my review, still remains within the realms of research rather than being considered appropriate for routine clinical practice.

Professor Christopher Chapple, B.Sc., M.D., F.R.C.S. (Urol), F.E.B.U.
Consultant Urological Surgeon, Royal Hallamshire Hospital
Honorary Senior Lecturer of Urology, University of Sheffield
Visiting Professor of Urology, Sheffield Hallam University
Adjunct Secretary General responsible for Education, European Association of Urology
Sheffield, UK

Professor Roger R. Dmochowski

Botulinum toxin use in urology has undergone substantial evolution over the last decade. Although not as yet approved in the majority of countries for indications in the lower urinary tract, rapid evidence is being accrued with appropriate levels of insight (randomized placebo controlled double blinded trials) which may meet regulatory criteria for approval for some lower urinary tract indications.

This book summarizes the evolution and journey of botulinum toxin in the management of lower urinary tract disease and is the work of two of the pre-eminent experts in the field of neurotoxin use in urology. The contribution of Michael Chancellor and Christopher Smith has not only been substantive from a clinical standpoint, but also from a mechanistic standpoint. Their studies have helped our understanding the actions of botulinum toxin on the lower urinary tract including affects on both afferent and efferent aspects of the reflexogenic activity of the lower urinary tract. Recent data would suggest that botulinum toxin has a complex mechanism of action, indeed affecting both aspects of the reflex arm controlling lower urinary tract function. Its role as an afferent modulator has only recently been appreciated and may underpin subsequent use of this toxin for an expanded group of indications in the lower urinary tract.

Questions regarding botulinum toxin use clinically remain legion. Appropriate dosing, administration, and patient selection being amongst the most problematic concerns; however, other issues related to repetitive administration such as potential changes within the lower urinary tract must be investigated as the medical community considers the use of botulinum toxin in the lower urinary tract.

As indicated in the table of contents this book summarizes essentially all of the lower urinary tract indications and reported uses of botulinum toxin. Again, for the majority of the world, these have not yet achieved regulatory approval, but ongoing studies exist across the areas indicated. Additionally, the book also summaries interesting uses of botulinum toxin (specifically neurogenic) and the health economic impact of this particular biologic entity which indeed may be substantive, at least initially. However, by reducing subsequent salvage related treatments costs, the overall impact may actually be beneficial.

The science of botulinum toxin no doubt will continue to evolve as experience with this toxin increases. More importantly, our ability to select or de-select groups of patients based upon primary pathology as causative for detrusor overactivity will clearly allow targeted use of not only botulinum toxin but other appropriate interventions for lower urinary tract disease. It is clear from this book, that the journey has started but is nowhere yet complete. As I read the contents of this book, I was reminded of Sir Isaac Newton's comments regarding the fact that all of us stand on the shoulders of those who go before us. The broad shoulders of Drs. Chancellor and Smith have clearly provided a foundation for the subsequent investigation and possible use of botulinum toxin in an expanded role for the lower urinary tract.

Roger R. Dmochowski, M.D.
Professor, Urologic Surgery
Director, Vanderbilt Continence Center
Director, Vanderbilt Female Reconstructive Fellowship
Executive Physician, Safety Vanderbilt University Adult Hospital
Nashville, Tennessee, USA

Professor Hann-Chorng Kuo

In this past decade, advances in functional urology have made great progress. Bench investigations have provided evidence for new clinical diagnosis and novel treatment options. Such progress has enabled physicians to revisit the traditional concept of lower urinary tract dysfunction, interstitial cystitis/painful bladder syndrome, and overactive bladder syndrome.

One of the most important advances achieved is the application of botulinum toxin for lower urinary tract dysfunction, which has allowed clinicians to effectively treat patients with neurogenic or non-neurogenic voiding dysfunctions and benign prostatic hyperplasia in high risk patients. I have witnessed reduction of prostatic volume and improvement of lower urinary tract symptoms as well as improved voiding function after prostatic botulinum toxin injections. In my experience, injecting 100 U onabotulinumtoxinA into the urethral sphincter not only can reduce the urethral resistance and facilitate spontaneous voiding, but also provide a chance of recovery of detrusor contractility in patients with idiopathic detrusor underactivity.

Decrease of bladder pain after botulinum toxin injection into the bladder also extends the therapeutic indication to interstitial cystitis/painful bladder syndrome (IC/PBS). Increased apoptosis and decreased proliferation of urothelium are recently found to be the possible pathophysiology of IC/PBS. These urothelial dysfunctions are closely linked to the chronic inflammation in IC/PBS. After botulinum toxin injection, we have found that maximal bladder capacity increases and the glomerulation grade after hydrodistension was reduced, suggesting the inflammation process was interrupted and that urothelial homeostasis was restored. Thus, intravesical botulinum toxin injection may reduce chronic inflammation of the bladder in IC/PBS, and improve bladder pain as well as increase bladder capacity. Botulinum toxin might play a role by eliminating central sensitization in IC/PBS. Repeated botulinum toxin injections may be necessary for symptom relief and long-term disease cure.

In my experience, intravesical injection with 100 U of onabotulinumtoxinA provides therapeutic effect on decreasing urgency incontinence episodes, urgency severity score and improved quality of life in patients with overactive bladder. I have noted that bladder base injection is as effective and safe as bladder body injection. However, high adverse event rates including dysuria, urinary tract infection, and acute urinary retention in the first one month remain problems, although they usually resolve by three months. Before one determines the appropriate dose, injecting sites, and depth of injection, careful patient selection is necessary. Informing the possible adverse events to patients who wish to be treated by botulinum toxin is mandatory before bladder injection for refractory overactive bladder. Nevertheless, the occurrence of adverse events has not influenced our final results and long-term success rate.

In the journey of botulinum toxin treatment of lower urinary tract dysfunctions, Michael Chancellor and Christopher Smith are the true pioneers. Their earliest works encourage many young researchers to devote themselves into this exciting field. The application of botulinum toxin in urology opens a window for urologists and urogynecologists to see an interesting garden.

Through the treatment results of more clinical trials, we learn more about how to apply botulinum toxin as a therapeutic agent in the treatment of lower urinary tract disorders. There are still many unknown phenomena of botulinum toxin treatment in lower urinary tract dysfunctions that deserve future investigation. The publication of this book provides a fundamental platform for the future research of botulinum toxin application in urology.

Hann-Chorng Kuo, M.D.
Professor and Chairman
Department of Urology
Buddhist Tzu Chi General Hospital and Tzu Chi University
Hualien, Taiwan

Introduction

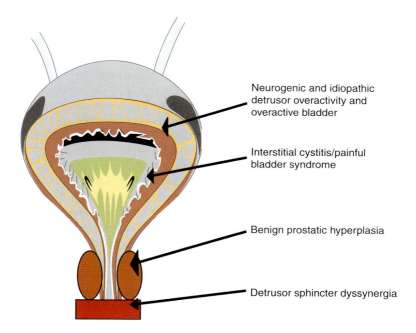

Since botulinum neurotoxin was initially approved for clinical use by the Food and Drug Administration in 1989, it has become a powerful therapeutic tool in the treatment of a variety of neurologic, ophthalmic, and other disorders manifested by abnormal, excessive, or inappropriate muscle contractions. The use of botulinum toxin has expanded to include gastrointestinal, orthopedic, dermatologic, secretory, cosmetic, and urinary tract disorders. Botulinum toxin has also been applied in the clinical management of pain in a number of areas, including myofascial pain disorders, migraine headache, low back pain, and other chronic pain syndromes including pain in the areas of the bladder, prostate, and the pelvic floor.

In using this practical book, we urge the health care professional to recognize the need for appropriate injection technique. This includes careful identification both of appropriate patients and of the muscles or regions that are to be injected, along with an awareness of the potential side effects of botulinum toxin therapy. We have included three appendices to highlight the practical operational nursing aspects of successfully and safely utilizing botulinum toxin in the urinary tract.

Tied to the successful use of botulinum toxin is the need to educate patients about the limitations of treatment, including the delay between treatment and the appearance of benefits, and the re-appearance of symptoms as the effects of botulinum toxin dissipate.

I started using botulinum toxin in 1998. I remember the frustration I felt back then having three female patients suffering from multiple sclerosis with high residual urine, recurrent urinary tract infections, and dyssynergia of the urethral sphincter. Nurse Margie O'Leary and me tried our best but were just unable to teach them to self-catheterize because of poor hand dexterity. After a consultation with the neurologists the patients were willing to try botulinum toxin instead of indwelling catheters or reconstructive surgery. The neurology clinic taught me how to prepare the toxin for injection and we went ahead with the procedure.

The procedures were uneventful and all three patients did very well after the sphincter botulinum injection. All three were able to void with significantly lower residual urine and there was no stress incontinence. I did some more research and discussed it with Professor William (Chet) de Groat at our lab meeting. Dr. de Groat was intrigued with the idea and recommended that we should pursue the study further in our lab. With de Groat's positive feedback I thought about bench top studies. At this time Christopher Smith started his National Institute of Health K12 Physician Scientist fellowship in Pittsburgh at the endorsement of his Mentor Dr. Tim Boone in Houston. Chris was looking for a new project to start and liked the concept of botulinum toxin research immediately. Working with Dr. George Somogyi, who led the neurotransmitter release and muscle contractility laboratory in the neurourology program, Chris and I quickly found that botulinum toxin not only effectively relaxed urethral strips but also detrusor muscle strips. We further found that botulinum toxin not only effectively blocked acetylcholine release from bladder and urethral strips but also norepinephrine release. Now this was something new and interesting.

As the cliché goes, the rest is history and led to a wonderful journey that started more than a decade ago since I took the first step.

We wish to express my most sincere gratitude to pioneers such as Dr. Dennis Dykstra and Professor Brigitte Schurch who opened up the field to urologists and urogynecologists.

Michael B. Chancellor, M.D.

Christopher P. Smith, M.D., M.B.A.

Acknowledgment

There are many other friends and colleagues who have helped us along the path from 1998 to today. Too many that we are sure to leave out important people. A few examples of additional people who worked directly with us include Chet de Groat, Naoki Yoshimura, George Somogyi, Piotr Radziszewski, Janet Erickson, Margie O'Leary, Sara Marx, Cindy Young, Darnetta Young, Tracy Cannon-Smith, Christopher Chermansky, Jill Bishoff, Timothy Boone, Alvaro Munoz, Mohit Khera, Pradeep Tyagi, Vikas Tyagi, Kenneth Peters, Ananias C. Diokno, Hsin-Tzu Liu, Wendy Leng, Teruhiko Yokoyama, Dae Kyung Kim, Hann-Chorng Kuo, Fernando de Miguel, Michele Anthony, Jonathan Kaufman, Maureen Cooney, Michelle Lajiness, Yao-Chi Chuang.

We are indebted to the experts from around the world whose help made urological development of botulinum toxin possible and for contributing to Chap. 11. We thank Professors Markus Naumann and Pankaj Jay Pasricha for sharing their perspectives on non-urological uses of toxin with genitourinary insight in Chap. 9. We appreciate very much Professor Yao-Chi Chuang's insight to the ideal BPH candidate for BoNT therapy in Chap. 8. Margie O'Leary, Michelle J. Lajiness and Mary Dierich were so wonderful with aiding us on the practical nursing appendixes. We want to especially thank Professors Christopher Chapple, Roger R. Dmochowski and Hann-Chorng Kuo for their friendship and writing a forward for our book. Thank you all.

We would finally like to thank our departments for their support for our research and our family for allowing us to take time out to write this book on an important topic we are passionate about.

Disclosure: Doctors Chancellor and Smith have both been consultants and investigators with the application of botulinum toxin in urology with Allergan, Inc Irvine California and have received financial compensation.

Michael B. Chancellor, M.D.

Christopher P. Smith, M.D., M.B.A.

Contents

Part I Rationale and Safety for BoNT

1. **Safety and General Principles of Botulinum Toxin Therapies: Pearls From Across Medical Fields** 3
   1.1 Introduction 3
   1.2 Considerations for the Safe Use of BoNT 3
   1.3 General Principles of Botulinum Toxin Therapy 6
   1.4 After BoNT Injection Patient Management Principles 7
   1.5 Storage and Dilution of Botulinum Toxins 8
       1.5.1 OnabotulinumtoxinA (BOTOX®) 8
       1.5.2 AbobotulinumtoxinA (Dysport®) 9
       1.5.3 RimabotulinumtoxinB (Myobloc and Neurobloc®) 10
       1.5.4 IncobotulinumtoxinA (Xeomin®) 10
   1.6 Issues in Multi-specialty Interactions 10
   1.7 Conclusions 11
   Reference 11

2. **Biology and Mechanism of Action** 13
   2.1 Introduction 13
   2.2 History of Medical Botulinum Toxin 13
   2.3 Seven Serotypes of Botulinum Toxin 14
   2.4 Pathophysiology 15
       2.4.1 Four Required Steps to Induce Paralysis 15
   2.5 BoNT Effect on Muscle Neurotransmission 17
   2.6 BoNT Action at Synapses and on Neuropeptides 18
   2.7 BoNT Action on Urinary Tract Striated and Smooth Muscles .. 18
       2.7.1 Efferent Effect 19
       2.7.2 Afferent Effect 20
       2.7.3 Effects on Acetylcholine and ATP Release 20
       2.7.4 Effect on Hot and Cold Sensitive Sensory Receptors .. 21
       2.7.5 Clinical Effects on Calcitonin Gene-Related Peptide and Substance P Release 21
       2.7.6 Inhibition of Nerve Growth Factor Release and Receptor Transport 22

2.8	Histological Impact of BoNT Injection	22
2.9	BoNT Antibody Production	23
2.10	Conclusion	24
References		25

Part II Bladder

3. Botulinum Toxin for Neurogenic Detrusor Overactivity 29
   3.1 Introduction 29
   3.2 Indications 29
        3.2.1 Spinal Cord Injury 30
        3.2.2 Multiple Sclerosis: Variable Spectrum and Disease Progression 31
        3.2.3 Pediatric Neurogenic Bladders 32
        3.2.4 Parkinson's Disease and Multisystem Atrophy 32
   3.3 What Is the Work-Up? 32
        3.3.1 History and Physical Examination 32
        3.3.2 Urodynamic Evaluation 33
   3.4 How to Do It 33
        3.4.1 Patient Preparation 33
        3.4.2 Cystoscope 36
        3.4.3 Botulinum Toxin Reconstitution 37
        3.4.4 Dose 38
        3.4.5 Depth, Location, and Amount of Injection 38
        3.4.6 Injection Technique 39
        3.4.7 Simultaneous Bladder and Sphincter BoNT Injection 41
        3.4.8 Post-procedure and Follow-Up 42
        3.4.9 How Long Does It Last and When Is Botulinum Toxin Injection Repeated 42
        3.4.10 Subsequent Dose Selection (Can You and Should You Go Up or Down on Dose) 43
        3.4.11 Risk of Antibody Formation 43
   3.5 What Are the Results 44
        3.5.1 Clinical Studies 44
        3.5.2 Duration of Effect 47
        3.5.3 Repeat Injections 47
        3.5.4 No Histological Damage to Bladder with BoNT Repeated Injections 49
        3.5.5 Can BoNT Improve Bladder Compliance? 49
        3.5.6 Adverse Events 52
        3.5.7 Simultaneous Bladder and Sphincter BoNT Injection 55
   3.6 Future Perspective: Electrical Neuromodulation and Stem Cell Research 56
   3.7 Conclusions 57
   References 57

4. Overactive Bladder and Idiopathic Detrusor Overactivity 61
    4.1 Introduction 61
    4.2 Rationale for BoNT Use in Idiopathic OAB 61
    4.3 How to Do It... 62
        4.3.1 Simplified Delivery Using Flexible Cystoscope 62
        4.3.2 Depth of Injection 64
    4.4 What Are the Results?...................................... 68
        4.4.1 Botulium Toxin Type A 68
        4.4.2 Botulinum Toxin Type B 70
        4.4.3 Predictors of Poor Response 71
    4.5 Side Effects 72
        4.5.1 Risk-Benefit Ratio 73
    4.6 Conclusions 76
    References 76

5. BoNT for Bladder and Pelvic Pain 79
    5.1 Introduction 79
    5.2 Indications 79
    5.3 What Is the Work-Up...................................... 80
        5.3.1 History and Physical Examination..................... 80
        5.3.2 Urodynamic Evaluation 80
    5.4 How to Do It... 81
        5.4.1 Patient Preparation................................ 81
        5.4.2 Cystoscope....................................... 81
        5.4.3 Botulinum Toxin Reconstitution 83
        5.4.4 Dose 83
        5.4.5 Depth, Location, and Amount of Injection 84
        5.4.6 Injection Technique 84
        5.4.7 Post-procedure and Follow-Up 85
        5.4.8 How Long Does It Last and When Is Botulinum
             Toxin Injection Repeated............................ 85
    5.5 What Are the Results 85
        5.5.1 Clinical Results IC/PBS............................. 85
        5.5.2 Chronic Female Pelvic Pain Syndromes 89
        5.5.3 Chronic Prostatis/Male Chronic Pelvic Pain Syndrome
             (CP/CPPS)....................................... 90
        5.5.4 Radiation and Inflammatory Cystitis 90
    5.6 Conclusions 91
    References 92

6. Pediatric Botulinum Toxin Applications 95
    6.1 Introduction 95
    6.2 Indications 96
        6.2.1 When to Consider Botulinum Toxin Injection........... 96
        6.2.2 Nonneurogenic Indications in Children................ 97
    6.3 What Is the Work-Up?..................................... 97

	6.3.1	History and Physical Examination	97
	6.3.2	Urodynamic Evaluation	97
6.4	How to Do It		98
	6.4.1	Cystoscope	98
	6.4.2	Botulinum Toxin Reconstitution	99
	6.4.3	Dose	99
	6.4.4	Depth, Location, and Amount of Injection	100
	6.4.5	Injection Technique	100
	6.4.6	Post-procedure and Follow-up	101
6.5	What Are the Results?		101
	6.5.1	Idiopathic Detrusor Overactivity Clinical Studies	104
	6.5.2	Voiding Dysfunction Clinical Studies	105
	6.5.3	Repeat Injection	106
6.6	Conclusions		106
References			107

Part III Prostate and Pelvic Floor

7. Botulinum Toxin Injection for Prostate Disorders 111

7.1	Introduction		111
7.2	Prostate BoNT Rationale and Mechanism of Action		113
7.3	Indications		115
	7.3.1	BPH	115
	7.3.2	Prostatitis/Prostatodynia	116
7.4	What Is the Work-up?		116
	7.4.1	History and Physical Examination	116
7.5	How to Do It		117
	7.5.1	BPH	117
	7.5.2	Prostatitis/Prostatodynia	121
7.6	What Are the Results?		121
	7.6.1	BPH	123
	7.6.2	Prostatitis/Prostatodynia	126
	7.6.3	Adverse Events	127
7.7	Conclusions		128
References			128

8. Sphincter and Pelvic Floor Disorders Applications 131

8.1	Introduction		131
	8.1.1	Detrusor-Sphincter Dyssynergia Pathology	131
8.2	Indications		132
	8.2.1	Neurogenic DSD	132
	8.2.2	Non-neurogenic DSD	133
	8.2.3	Pelvic Floor and Pain	134
8.3	What Is the Work-Up		134
	8.3.1	History and Physical Examination	134
	8.3.2	Urodynamic Evaluation	134

	8.4	How to Do It	137
	8.4.1	Neurogenic DSD	137
	8.4.2	Simultaneous Bladder and Sphincter BoNT Injection	138
	8.4.3	Non-neurogenic DSD	138
	8.4.4	Pelvic Floor and Pain	139
	8.5	What Are the Results	141
	8.5.1	Neurogenic DSD	142
	8.5.2	Adverse Events	144
	8.5.3	Simultaneous Bladder and Sphincter BoNT Injection	145
	8.5.4	Non-neurogenic DSD	145
	8.5.5	Post-surgical Retention	146
	8.5.6	Bladder Neck Dyssynergia (Primary Bladder Neck Obstruction)	147
	8.5.7	Pelvic Floor and Pain	147
	8.5.8	Pain Due to Hypertonic Pelvic Floor Muscles	148
	8.5.9	Vulvodynia	149
	8.5.10	Chronic Prostatitis/Male Chronic Pelvic Pain Syndrome	149
	8.6	Conclusion	150
		References	150

Part VI Role of BoNT in Medicine

9. Non-urological Uses of Toxin with Genitourinary Insight 155
    9.1 Introduction 155
    9.2 BoNT in Pain Syndromes 155
        9.2.1 Back Pain 155
        9.2.2 Myofascial Pain Syndromes......................... 156
        9.2.3 Headache and Migraine 158
    9.3 BoNT in the Gastrointestinal Tract 159
        9.3.1 Achalasia 160
        9.3.2 Chronic Anal Fissure 161
        9.3.3 Emerging Gastrointestinal Uses of BoNT Therapy 162
    9.4 BoNT for Hyperhidrosis 163
        9.4.1 Therapeutic Approaches for Hyperhidrosis 163
        9.4.2 The Role of BoNT in Hyperhidrosis Treatment 163
        9.4.3 Clinical Studies of BoNT: Axillary Hyperhidrosis 164
        9.4.4 Clinical Studies of BoNT: Palmar Hyperhidrosis 165
        9.4.5 BoNT for Drooling................................. 165
    9.5 Conclusions 166
    References 166

10. Health Economics of Botulinum Toxin Application 169
    10.1 Introduction 169
    10.2 Sacral Nerve Neuromodulation 169
        10.2.1 Clinical Results with Sacral Nerve Neuromodulation 170

10.3	Comparative Cost Analysis	170
	10.3.1 Results	170
10.4	Other Recent Reports	172
	10.4.1 BoNT Versus Anticholinergics	172
	10.4.2 BoNT Versus Augmentation Cystoplasty	172
	10.4.3 Different Brands of Botulinum Toxin	173
	10.4.4 BoNT Cost to the French Health Care System	173
	10.4.5 BoNT Versus New Modalities	174
10.5	Conclusion	174
	References	175

11. Perspectives from Around the World: Panorama of Where We Are and Where We Are Going 177
    11.1   Australia: Jeffrey Thavaseelan 177
    11.2   Belgium: Dirk De Ridder 178
    11.3   Canada: Sender Herschorn 179
    11.4   France: Emmanuel Chartier-Kastler 180
    11.5   Germany: Tim Schneider 181
    11.6   Indian: Sanjay Pandey 181
            11.6.1 Early Years of BoNT in Indian Urology (2005–2007) .. 181
            11.6.2 The BoNT "Wonder Years" in Indian Urology (2008–2010) 182
            11.6.3 Challenges and Drafts for Future (2011 – Beyond) 183
    11.7   Italy: Antonella Giannantoni 183
    11.8   Japan: Yukio Homma 184
    11.9   Korea: Kyu-Sung Lee 185
    11.10 The Netherlands: John Heesakkers 186
    11.11 Portugal: Francisco Cruz 187
    11.12 Singapore: Michael Wong 188
    11.13 Taiwan: Alex T.L. Lin 189
    11.14 United Kingdom: Arun Sahai and Prokar Dasgupta 190
    11.15 United Kingdom Urogynaecology: Anga S. Arunkalaivanan 191
    References 192

Appendix 1 195
Appendix 2 199
Appendix 3 201

Index 205

Part I
Rationale and Safety for BoNT

Safety and General Principles of Botulinum Toxin Therapies: Pearls From Across Medical Fields

1.1 Introduction

Since the initial trials and approval of the medicinal use of botulinum toxin in the 1980s, therapeutic applications of botulinum neurotoxins have come from virtually every medical specialty. Table 1.1 is a list of applications of botulinum toxin (BoNT) and the list continues to expand. In this chapter, we hope to summarize some of the general treatment principles that have been learned from other specialties, especially neurology and rehabilitation medicine who both have been using BoNT for much longer than urologists and gynecologists, in order to help us better treat our patients.

1.2 Considerations for the Safe Use of BoNT

Healthcare professionals should be aware that a boxed warning has been added to the prescribing information of BoNT in the United States to highlight that BoNT can spread from the area of injection to produce symptoms consistent with botulism. Box 1.1 summarizes general notices by public health officials on key facts regarding botulism. The US Food and Drug Administration (FDA) in 2009 issued a new warning that botulinum toxin must carry warning labels explaining that the material has the potential to spread from the injection site to distant parts of the body – with the risk of serious difficulties, like problems with swallowing or breathing.

Symptoms of botulism include unexpected loss of strength or muscle weakness, hoarseness or trouble talking (dysphonia), trouble saying words clearly (dysarthria), loss of bladder control, trouble breathing, trouble swallowing, double vision, blurred vision, and drooping eyelids.

Swallowing and breathing difficulties can be life-threatening and there have been reports of deaths related to the effect of spread of BoNT. Be aware that children treated for spasticity are at greatest risk of these symptoms, but symptoms can also occur in adults treated for spasticity and other conditions. Realize that cases of toxin

Table 1.1 Expanding therapeutic applications of botulinum neurotoxin

Focal dystonias
- Blepharospasm
- Oromandibular-facial-lingual dystonia
- Cervical dystonia
- Laryngeal dystonia (spasmodic dysphonia)
- Focal dystonias: involuntary, sustained, or spasmodic patterned muscle activity
- Task-specific dystonia (occupational cramps, e.g., writer's cramps and other limb dystonias)
- Other focal dystonias

Other involuntary movements
- Voice, head, and limb tremor
- Palatal myoclonus
- Hemifacial spasm
- Tics

Other inappropriate contractions
- Smooth muscle hyperactive disorders of the gastrointestinal and genitourinary systems
- Strabismus
- Nystagmus
- Stuttering
- Painful rigidity
- Temporomandibular joint disorders associated with increased muscle activity
- Muscle contraction headaches
- Lumbosacral strain and back spasms
  - Radiculopathy with secondary muscle spasm
- Spasticity (e.g., stroke, head injury, paraplegia, cerebral palsy, multiple sclerosis)
- Achalasia
- Urinary sphincter dyssynergia
- Pelvic and rectal spasms (anismus, vaginismus)
- Achalasia cardia
- Hirschsprung disease
- Sphincter of Oddi dysfunctions
- Following hemorrhoidectomy
- Chronic anal fissures

Other applications
- Protective ptosis
- Sweating disorders
- Axillary and palmar hyperhidrosis
- Frey syndrome, also known as auriculotemporal syndrome (gustatory sweating of the cheek after parotid surgery)
- Cosmetic
- Hyperkinetic facial lines (glabellar frown lines, crow's feet)
- Genitourinary track dysfunctions including bladder and prostate
- Migraine and tension headache
- Pain
- Myofascial pain syndrome

spread have occurred at BoNT doses comparable to those used to treat cervical dystonia and at lower doses.

Botulinum toxin products and brands are not interchangeable and the established drug names of the BoNT products have been changed to emphasize the differing dose to potency ratios of these products. The potency of each toxin is expressed in units of activity. Although there are similarities among the commercial preparations of BoNT, they have different doses, efficacy and safety profiles, and should not be considered generic equivalents comparable by single dose ratios. In other words, the doses expressed in units are not comparable from one BoNT product to the next (i.e., units of one product cannot be converted into units of another product). We will review the commercially available toxins in this chapter.

> **Box 1.1: Essentials of Human Botulism**
> Human botulism is a rare but very serious disease. Botulism is mainly a food borne intoxication but it can also be transmitted through wound infections. The bacterium Clostridium botulinum is the same bacterium that is used to produce pharmaceutical botulinum toxin. What is used in medical BoNT is the toxin alone in small doses.
>
> **Symptoms**
> Incidence of botulism is low, but the mortality rate is high if treatment is not immediate and proper. The disease can be fatal in 5–10% of cases.
>
> Food borne botulism occurs when the organism *Clostridium botulinum* is allowed to grow and produce toxin in food which is then eaten without sufficient cooking to inactivate the toxin. *Clostridium botulinum* is an anaerobic bacterium. This happens most often in lightly preserved foods such as fermented, salted or smoked fish, and meat products and in inadequately processed home canned or home bottled low acid foods such as vegetables. The food traditionally implicated differs between countries and will reflect local eating habits and food preservation procedures.
>
> Botulism symptoms are not caused by the organism itself, but by the toxin that the bacterium releases. They usually appear within 12–36 h after exposure.
>
> The characteristic early symptoms and signs are marked fatigue, weakness, and vertigo, usually followed by blurred vision, dry mouth, and difficulty in swallowing and speaking.
>
> Vomiting, diarrhea, constipation, and abdominal swelling may occur. The disease can progress to weakness in the neck and arms, after which the respiratory muscles and muscles of the lower body are affected. The paralysis may make breathing difficult. There is no fever and no loss of consciousness.
>
> Similar symptoms usually appear in individuals who shared the same food. Most patients recover, if given proper and immediate treatment, including prompt diagnosis, early administration of antitoxin, and intensive respiratory care.

Treatment
Antitoxin administration is indicated as soon as possible after the clinical diagnosis of botulism has been made. Severe botulism cases require supportive treatment, especially mechanical ventilation, which may be required for weeks or months. Antibiotics are not required (except in the case of wound botulism). There is a vaccine against botulism, but it is rarely used as its effectiveness has not been fully evaluated.

If exposure to the toxin via an aerosol is suspected, in order to prevent additional exposure to the patient and health care providers, the clothing of the patient must be removed and stored in plastic bags until it can be washed with soap and water. The patient must shower thoroughly. Food and water samples associated with suspect cases must be obtained immediately, stored in proper sealed containers, and sent to reference laboratories in order to help prevent further cases.

Prevention
Prevention of botulism is based on good hygiene and food preparation practices. Botulism may be prevented by inactivation of the bacterial spores in heat-sterilized, canned products, or by inhibiting growth in all other products.

Commercial heat pasteurization (vacuum packed pasteurized products, hot smoked products) may not be sufficient to kill all spores and therefore safety of these products must be based on preventing growth and toxin production. Refrigeration temperatures combined with salt content or acidic conditions will prevent the growth of toxin.

1.3 General Principles of Botulinum Toxin Therapy

- The physician should review the known side effects of BoNT treatment for the specific product to be used – including possible headache, rash, bruising, or muscle weakness – with the patient and obtain informed consent.
- BoNT therapy should be individualized according to specific patient needs and the muscles or organ affected, and the patient should be prepared with respect to what he or she is likely to experience after the injection.
- The equipment needs will vary according to the anatomic target for injection.
- For pelvic floor muscles, as with large muscle groups in other applications, such as the hamstrings, a 1 in. or 1.5 in., 25 gauge needle is adequate. A 1.0 mL tuberculin-type syringe with a 5/8 in., 25 gauge needle is adequate for superficial muscles or trigger pain and vulvodynia. Transurethral approach to the bladder, sphincter, and percutaneous approach to the prostate will be discussed in following specific chapters.
- Outside of our field, the use of electromyography guidance or electrical stimulation has been advocated to identify specific muscles – particularly smaller muscles. For muscles requiring electromyography guidance, a cannulated monopolar

Table 1.2 Principles of treatment plan for BoNT therapy
- *Diagnosis and baseline assessment*
- *Specific symptoms*
- *Co-morbid conditions*
- *Patient expectations*
  – Patient needs and goals
  – Reduce or discontinue use of acute pain medications
  – Decreased intensity of symptoms and/or pain
  – Improved function and reduced dysfunction
  – Increased intensity of physical therapy and rehabilitation
- *Patient education*
  – Goals of therapy
  – Purpose of each component of the treatment plan
  – Importance of follow-up evaluation and care
  – Potential side effects

    needle cathode, through which BoNT can be injected, is used. Surface reference (anode) and ground electrodes should be placed near the cathode needle. Electromyography may be helpful for pelvic floor sphincter injection.
- After the patient is placed in a position where the desired muscle can be targeted, BoNT can then be given after aspiration to prevent intravascular injection.
- Use of operating rooms or special procedure (sterile) rooms equipped with monitoring devices is not necessary in the vast majority of cases.
- Before initiating BoNT treatment, the physician and patient should develop a treatment plan (Table 1.2), including a baseline assessment of the severity of pain and disability, setting goals for treatment, and establishing appropriate expectations for treatment outcome as well as postinjection rehabilitation.

1.4 After BoNT Injection Patient Management Principles

- Patients do not require prolonged observation in the immediate postinjection period; 10–15 min is adequate for most patients. Wheals may be visible at the injection sites, but patients should be reassured that these will disappear within a couple of hours.
- Patients should be re-evaluated 2–4 weeks postinjection. This may only be necessary after the first injection. Patients should be advised with the use of acute medications, if necessary, for pain management.
- Patients should also be prepared for the likely time course of the effect of BoNT therapy, which may take several weeks to reach peak efficacy. The duration of the clinical effect is roughly 12 weeks in some cases of skeletal muscle injection but can last 9–12 months with bladder and prostate injections.
- For patients with spasticity and a variety of neuromuscular pain disorders, adjunctive physical therapy and rehabilitation helps to restore the balance

Table 1.3 Guidelines for BoNT treatment

- Consider if BoNT therapy is appropriate for the patient and condition being treated
- Determine which muscles need to be injected
- Use the smallest effective total dose and volume
- Determine the appropriate dosage and the number and volume of injections per session
- Use appropriate techniques to achieve precise injection and reduce the risk of complications
- Follow-up with the patient to assess efficacy, safety, and satisfaction with treatment
- Record details of treatment (dose, volume, sites) and patient response to treatment to guide future injections
- Administer subsequent injection with as long an inter dose interval as possible
- Reassess the treatment regiment and the patient's response

between muscles working as a coordinated, functional unit. The muscle relaxation induced by BoNT and the reduction in pain provide an opportunity to intensify the physical therapy regimen.
- Table 1.3 provides a global summary of guidelines for the management of patients receiving BoNT therapy.

1.5 Storage and Dilution of Botulinum Toxins

Although there are seven serotypes of botulinum toxin, only types A and B are in clinical use. The potency of each toxin is expressed in units of activity. The different preparations have different doses, efficacy and safety profiles, and should not be considered generic equivalents comparable by single dose ratios. Three of the commonly used botulinum toxins are serotype A while only one (i.e., rimabotulinumtoxinB, Myobloc®) is serotype B. Albanese (2011) recently presented a new terminology for preparations of botulinum neurotoxins and Table 1.4 lists botulinum toxins currently marketed.
- AbobotulinumtoxinA (Dysport; Ipsen Ltd., Berkshire, UK)
- IncobotulinumtoxinA (Xeomin; Merz Pharmaceuticals GmbH. Germany)
- OnabotulinumtoxinA (Botox and Botox Cosmetic, Allergan, Inc., Irvine, CA)
- RimabotulinumtoxinB (Myobloc and Neurobloc; US WorldMeds, Louisville, KY)

1.5.1 OnabotulinumtoxinA (BOTOX®)

- Vacuum dried onabotulinumtoxinA (onaBoNT-A) is available in vials containing 100 units of onabotulinumtoxinA. One vial (100 units) is diluted with varying amounts of preservative-free 0.9% saline according to the site of injection.
- Some investigators suggest the use of saline with preservative. It has been shown to be effective in cosmesis, with less pain on injection.

1.5 Storage and Dilution of Botulinum Toxins

Table 1.4 Botulinum toxins currently marketed

Serotype	A	A	A	B
Generic name	*Onabotulinumtoxin*A	*Abobotulinumtoxin*A	*Incobotulinumtoxin*A	*Rimabotulinumtoxin*B
Brand name	Botox	Dysport	Xeomin	Myobloc/Neurobloc[a]
Manufacturer	Allergan Inc (United States)	Ipsen (France)	Merz pharmaceuticals GmbH (Germany)	US WorldMeds (United States)
Packaging, U/vial	100	500	100	2,500, 5,000, or 10,000
Preparation	Dry: vacuum dried	Dry: lyophilized	Dry: lyophilized	Solution (5,000 U/mL)
Storage of packaged product	−5°C or 2–8°C	Room temperature	Room temperature	2–8°C
Storage after reconstitution	2–8°C for 24 h	2–8°C for several hours	2–8°C for 24 h	For a few hours
Specific activity, U/ng	20	40	167	75–125

[a]Myobloc is the brand name in the United States, Canada, and Korea. Neurobloc is the brand name in the European Union, Iceland, and Norway

- Because the product and diluent usually do not contain a preservative, the reconstituted onabotulinumtoxinA should be used within 24 h. During this time, the BoNT should be refrigerated at 2–8°C.
- The potency of onaBoNT-A is measured in mouse units. One mouse unit of onaBoNT-A is equivalent to the amount of toxin that will kill 50% of a group of 20 g Swiss-Webster mice within 3 days of intraperitoneal injection (lethal dose in 50% [LD50]).
- LD50 of onaBoNT-A for a 70-kg adult male has been calculated to be 2,500–3,000 U (35–40 U/kg).

1.5.2 AbobotulinumtoxinA (Dysport®)

- Lyophilized abobotulinumtoxinA is available in vials of 500 U. It should be stored at 2–8°C at the facility where it is to be used.
- Some investigators suggest the use of saline with preservative. It has been shown to be effective in cosmesis, with less pain on injection.
- Because the product does not contain an antimicrobial agent, it is recommended that the reconstituted abobotulinumtoxinA be used immediately after reconstitution, although the reconstituted abobotulinumtoxinA may be stored at 2–8°C for up to 8 h before use.
Reloxin/Dysport: Medicis Pharmaceutical Corporation of Scottsdale, licensed from Ipsen. Seeking US approval; approved in Europe for non-cosmetic purposes under the brand name Dysport.

1.5.3 RimabotulinumtoxinB (Myobloc and Neurobloc®)

- RimabotulinumtoxinB, the only serotype B botulinum toxin commercially available, is shipped as a refrigerated, liquid formulation, which may be further diluted (with normal saline).
- RimabotulinumtoxinB is provided as a sterile injectable solution at a concentration of 5,000 U/mL and a pH of 5.5. Vials contain 0.5 mL (2,500 U), 1.0 mL (5,000 U), or 2.0 mL (10,000 U). Because vials are overfilled, each vial contains slightly more toxin than these indicated volumes.
- Vials of rimabotulinumtoxinB may be stored at 2–8°C for up to 21 months. To preserve the integrity of the toxin, vials should not be frozen or shaken. RimabotulinumtoxinB may be diluted with sterile saline (without preservative). Since the volume in the vials is greater than the nominal volume, dilution should be performed in the syringe and not in the vial. Diluted toxin should be used within 4 h.
- Minimum lethal dose of rimabotulinumtoxinB in monkeys is 2,400 U/kg.

US WorldMeds of Louisville, KY acquired Solstice Neurosciences, Inc in August 2010 and have rights to RimabotulinumtoxinB. Some experts have noticed shorter duration of clinical activity with rimabotulinumtoxinB versus botulinum toxin serotype A. We generally reserve rimabotulinumtoxinB in cases where patient form antibodies to and are not responding clinically to serotype A toxin treatment.

1.5.4 IncobotulinumtoxinA (Xeomin®)

Mertz is a German pharmaceutical company that is manufacturing IncobotulinumtoxinA (Xeomin®) as the third botulinum toxin serotype A licensed in the United Kingdom. IncobotulinumtoxinA is an innovative botulinum toxin formulation in which the complexing proteins have been removed by an extensive purification process from the botulinum toxin complex.

In contrast to the other commercially available preparations, incobotulinumtoxinA only contains the pure 150 kD neurotoxin. It is widely accepted that the bacterial protein present in other products play a role as promoters of an immune reaction, resulting in a loss of effect and reduction in duration of activity. IncobotulinumtoxinA, without the complexing proteins, appear to have the lowest content of protein of the available botulinum toxins and repeated application of incobotulinumtoxinA has minimal risk of neutralizing antibody formation.

1.6 Issues in Multi-specialty Interactions

Regulatory agencies are likely to approve the use of onabotulinumtoxinA for the indication of neurogenic detrusor overactivity. This raises the likelihood that botulinum toxin may be used by urologists and urogynecologists in addition to neurologists and rehabilitation medicine specialists for the treatment of multiple conditions in the same patient.

What treating physicians need to know is that experts with botulinum toxin suggest same day treatments for multiple indications to minimize immunogenicity. Without formal guidelines we believe that a wait period between multi-specialty treatments of 8–12 weeks seems reasonable. In other words, if a patient recently received injection by her neurologist for spasticity, the urologist or urogynecologist should wait 8–12 weeks before bladder injection for neurogenic detrusor overactivity. Furthermore, we suggest avoiding product combinations in the same patient.

1.7 Conclusions

It is important to remember that botulinum toxin products and brands are not interchangeable and the established drug names of the BoNT products have been changed to emphasize the differing dose to potency ratios of these products. The potency of each toxin is expressed in units of activity. Although there are similarities among the commercial preparations of BoNT, they have different doses, efficacy, and safety profiles, and should not be considered generic equivalents comparable by single dose ratios. In other words, the doses expressed in units are not comparable from one BoNT product to the next (i.e., units of one product cannot be converted into units of another product).

Reference

Albanese A (2011) Terminology of preparations of botulinum neurotoxins. What a difference a name makes. JAMA 305:89–90

Biology and Mechanism of Action

2.1 Introduction

Since botulinum neurotoxin was initially approved in 1989 by the U.S. Food and Drug Administration, it has become a powerful therapeutic tool in the treatment of a variety of neurologic, ophthalmic and other disorders.

The use of botulinum toxin (BoNT) has expanded to include gastrointestinal, orthopedic, dermatologic, secretory, and cosmetic disorders. BoNT has also been applied in the clinical management of pain in a number of areas, including myofascial pain disorders, migraine headache, low back pain, and other chronic pain syndromes. Most exciting is the promising results of botulinum toxin use in a variety of genitourinary organs and lower urinary track dysfunctions.

Botulinum neurotoxins are well known for their ability to potently and selectively disrupt and modulate neurotransmission. Only recently have urologists become interested in the potential use of BoNT in patients with detrusor overactivity and other urological disorders. We will review mechanisms by which BoNT modulates acetylcholine and other biochemical messengers at presynaptic nerve terminals in the detrusor smooth muscle and possibly the urothelium. We will also review what is known about potentially important non-cholinergic mechanisms modulating the function of detrusor smooth muscle and bladder afferent sensory processing.

2.2 History of Medical Botulinum Toxin

The Sausage Poison: The German physician and poet Justinus Kerner (1786–1862) first developed the idea of a possible therapeutic use of botulinum toxin, which he called "sausage poison."

1870, Muller (another German physician) coined the name botulism. The Latin form is botulus, which means sausage.

1895, Professor Emile Van Ermengem, of Belgium, first isolated the bacterium Clostridium botulinum.

1928, Dr. Herman Sommer first isolated purified form of botulinum toxin type A (BoNT-A) as a stable acid precipitate.

1946, Dr. Edward J Schantz succeeded in purifying BoNT-A in crystalline form–cultured Clostridium botulinum and isolated the toxin.

1950s, Dr. Vernon Brooks discovered that when BoNT-A is injected into a hyperactive muscle, it blocks the release of acetylcholine from motor nerve endings.

1973, Dr. Alan B. Scott, of Smith-Kettlewell Eye Research Institute, used BoNT-A in monkey experiments.

1980, Dr. Scott used BoNT-A for the first time in humans to treat strabismus.

1989, OnabotulinumtoxinA (Botox®; Botox Cosmetic®, Allergan, Inc., Irvine, CA) was approved by the US Food and Drug Administration (FDA) for the treatment of strabismus, blepharospasm, and hemifacial spasm in patients aged younger than 12 years.

The acceptance of BoNT-A use for the treatment of spasticity and muscle pain disorders is growing. The clinical use of botulinum toxin serotype B, RimabotulinumtoxinB (Myobloc®; Elan Pharmaceuticals, Inc., Princeton, NJ), has been studied. RimabotulinumtoxinB was approved by the FDA in 2000, for treatment of cervical dystonia, to reduce the severity of abnormal head position and neck pain.

Use of BoNT-F also is under investigation in patients who have become immunologically resistant to serotypes A and B.

2.3 Seven Serotypes of Botulinum Toxin

Seven botulinum toxin serotypes (A, B, C [C1 and C2], D, E, F, and G) are produced by Clostridium botulinum, a gram-positive anaerobic bacterium. The clinical syndrome of botulism can occur following ingestion of contaminated food, from colonization of the infant gastrointestinal tract, or from a wound infection. Human botulism is caused mainly by types A, B, E, and (rarely) F. Types C and D cause toxicity only in animals. All of these serotypes inhibit acetylcholine release, although their intracellular target proteins, the characteristics of their actions, and their potencies vary substantially (Fig. 2.1).

The various botulinum toxins possess individual potencies, and care is required to assure proper use and avoid medication errors. Recent changes to the established drug names by the FDA were intended to reinforce these differences and prevent medication errors. The products and their approved indications include the following:

- OnabotulinumtoxinA (Botox, Botox Cosmetic)
  - Botox – Cervical dystonia, severe primary axillary hyperhidrosis, strabismus, blepharospasm, chronic migraine
  - Botox Cosmetic – Moderate-to-severe glabellar lines
- AbobotulinumtoxinA (Dysport) – Cervical dystonia, moderate-to-severe glabellar lines
- IncobotulinumtoxinA (Xeomin) – Cervical dystonia, blepharospasm
- Rimabotulinumtoxin B (Myobloc) – Cervical dystonia

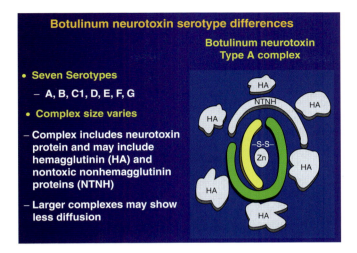

Fig. 2.1 Seven immunologically distinct serotypes of botulinum toxin (types A, B, C1, D, E, F, and G). The neurotoxin protein complexes formed by the various serotypes vary in size from ≈300 kD to ≈900 kD. The complexes include the neurotoxin protein and may include hemagglutinin (*HA*) and nontoxic, nonhemagglutinin (*NTNH*) proteins. The smallest complex formed includes the neurotoxin and a NTNH protein. The largest complex formed includes the neurotoxin and both NTNH and HA proteins

2.4 Pathophysiology

Botulinum toxins are synthesized as single chain polypeptides with a molecular weight of around 150 kDa (DasGupta 1994). Initially, the parent chain is cleaved into its active, dichain polypeptide form consisting of a heavy chain (approx. 100 kDa) connected by a disulfide bond to a light chain (approx. 50 kDa) with an associated zinc atom (Schiavo et al. 1992).

2.4.1 Four Required Steps to Induce Paralysis

1. Binding of the toxin heavy chain to a specific nerve terminal receptor
2. Internalization of the toxin within the nerve terminal
3. Translocation of the light-chain into the cytosol
4. Inhibition of neurotransmitter release

Neurotransmitter release involves the ATP-dependent transport of the vesicle from the cytosol to the plasma membrane (Barinaga 1993). Vesicle docking requires the interaction of various cytoplasmic, vesicle, and target membrane (i.e., SNARE: soluble N-ethylmaleimide-sensitive fusion attachment protein receptor) proteins, some of which are specifically targeted with clostridial neurotoxins (Fig. 2.2; Table 2.1). BoNT-A, for example, cleaves the cytosolic translocation protein SNAP-25, thus preventing vesicle fusion with the plasma membrane (Schiavo et al. 1993).

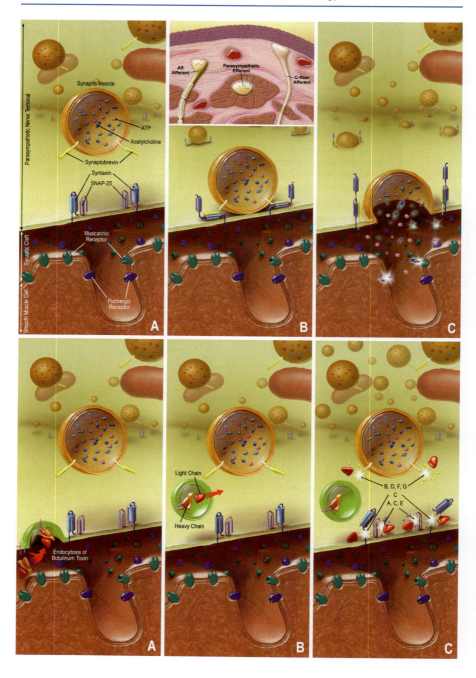

Table 2.1 Botulinum toxin types, target sites, discoverers, and year discovered

Type	Target	Discoverer	Year
A	SNAP-25	Landman	1904
B	VAMP	Ermengem	1897
C1	Syntaxin	Bengston and Seldon	1922
D	VAMP	Robinson	1929
E	SNAP-25	Gunnison	1936

Recent studies have identified the binding site for the BoNT-A heavy chain C-terminus to be a synaptic vesicle protein called SV2 (Dong et al. 2006). SV2 is a synaptic vesicle protein on the surface of nerve terminals that may increase when more neurotransmitter is released. This allows BoNT-A to preferentially target nerves that are more active. Expression of SV2 may also be inhibited by BoNT-A intoxication, which allows remaining extracellular toxin to bind to and inhibit, unoccupied nerve terminals to induce a greater paralytic effect.

Recovery occurs through proximal axonal sprouting and muscle re-innervation by formation of a new neuromuscular junction or the original neuromuscular junction regenerates.

- BoNT-A and BoNT-E cleave synaptosome-associated protein (SNAP-25), a presynaptic membrane protein required for fusion of neurotransmitter-containing vesicles.
- BoNT-B, BoNT-D, and BoNT-F cleave a vesicle-associated membrane protein (VAMP), also known as synaptobrevin.
- BoNT-C acts by cleaving syntaxin, a target membrane protein and SNAP-25.

2.5 BoNT Effect on Muscle Neurotransmission

BoNT is synthesized as a biologically inactive single-chain polypeptide (molecular mass ~150 kDa) that is activated by proteolytic cleavage of the polypeptide chain

Fig. 2.2 Top 3 Panels: Schematic diagram demonstrating normal fusion and release of acetylcholine from nerve terminals via interaction of vesicle and membrane bound (SNARE) proteins: **A)** nerve terminal in an unactivated state displaying numerous vesicles containing the neurotransmitter acetylcholine; **B)** following nerve activation, assembly of the SNARE protein complex (e.g., synaptobrevin, SNAP-25, and syntaxin) occurs that leads to; **C)** release of acetylcholine and activation of postjunctional muscarinic receptors, resulting in bladder contraction. Bottom 3 panels: **A)** binding of the toxin heavy chain to nerve terminal receptor and internalization of the toxin within the nerve terminal; **B)** translocation of the light-chain into the cytosol and; **C)** inhibition of neurotransmitter release by cleavage of specific SNARE proteins (A-G represent different botulinum toxin serotypes). (Copyright obtained from Smith and Chancellor 2004)

into a 100-kDa heavy chain and a 50-kDa light chain linked by a disulfide bond (Aoki 2005). The heavy chain is involved in the binding of the neurotoxin into specific parts of the peripheral nervous system and in the transport of the neurotoxin into the neuronal cytosol, while the light chain is responsible for cleavage of the intracellular protein chain transporting acetylcholine vesicles into the synaptic cleft (Dolly et al. 1984).

BoNT, taken up into the nerve terminals, cleaves the SNARE proteins, preventing assembly of the fusion complex and thus blocking the release of Acetycholine (ACh), leading to relaxation of the muscle. BoNT-A cleaves synaptosome-associated proteins of 25 kDa (SNAP-25) (Blasi et al. 1993), whereas BoNT-B cleaves vesicle-associated membrane protein (VAMP), also known as synaptobrevin.

Injection of BoNT into a muscle reduces alpha motoneuron activity on the extrafusal muscle fibers. Muscle spindles are simultaneously inhibited by the toxin's blockade of the motoneuron control of intrafusal fibers and by its subsequent reduction of afferent signaling, thereby reducing feedback to the motoneurons and other pathways to reduce muscle contraction.

2.6 BoNT Action at Synapses and on Neuropeptides

In preclinical studies, BoNT therapy also leads to altered afferent input to the central nervous system produced by the effect on muscle spindles. The release of substance P, a neuropeptide involved in neurogenic inflammation and the genesis of pain disorders, also requires the SNARE protein activity that is inhibited by BoNT (Aoki 2005). In other preclinical studies, BoNT has also been shown to suppress the release of glutamate, another neurotransmitter involved in nociception in the periphery and in the dorsal horn of the spinal cord (Cui et al. 2004). Moreover, BoNT can reduce the release of other neurotransmitters (Ashton and Dolly 1988) and neuromediators, including epinephrine, norepinephrine, and calcitonin gene-related peptide.

While BoNT appears to have no direct central nervous system activity, its effects on the neuromuscular junction and muscle spindle organs may have indirect central nervous system effects. At the spinal level, BoNT produces reflex inhibition of motoneurons and subsequent afferent input suppression.

On the supraspinal level, BoNT normalizes altered intracortical inhibition and somatosensory evoked potentials. Positron emission tomography scans of writer's cramp patients treated with BoNT found that treatment resulted in enhanced activation of parietal cortex and motor accessory areas but failed to improve the impaired activation of the primary motor cortex seen in the condition (Gilio et al. 2000).

2.7 BoNT Action on Urinary Tract Striated and Smooth Muscles

None of the clinically available Clostridial neurotoxins cause death of neurons or myocytes, or alteration of other cellular constituents. Thus, these neurotoxins are not toxic to tissues. Rather, in muscles, they act as biochemical neuromodulators, temporarily inactivating cholinergic transmission at the neuromuscular junction. Historically, the molecular mechanisms of BoNT have mostly been elucidated in studies of striated muscle. More recently, as a result of recognizing new clinical applications of BoNT, there have been studies conducted on the biological effects of BoNT on smooth muscle (Atiemo et al. 2005).

Despite some apparent differences at the cellular level, BoNT administration has the same clinical effect on both smooth and striated muscle. In the case of BoNT administration to the bladder wall, there is an increase in bladder capacity, with a reduction in incontinence episodes and symptoms of urgency. A more complete neuromuscular blockade of the detrusor results in impaired voiding and/or urinary retention if relatively larger doses of BoNT are used (Schurch et al. 2005).

2.7.1 Efferent Effect

Smith and colleagues found significant decrease in the release of labeled acetylcholine in BoNT injected in normal rat bladders suggesting that BoNT could reduce cholinergic nerve induced bladder activity (Smith et al. 2003a) (Fig. 2.3). Although BoNT is known to exhibit cholinergic specificity, release of other transmitters can be inhibited, particularly if adequate concentrations are utilized. For example, contractile data suggests that BoNT may impair ATP release in addition to acetylcholine release from isolated bladder tissue (Smith et al. 2003b). Datta and associates (2010) recently demonstrated decreased muscarinic receptor levels were restored back to control levels in the urothelium and suburothelium of patients successfully treated with BoNT for neurogenic and idiopathic detrusor overactivity.

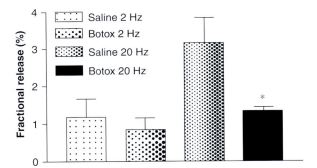

Fig. 2.3 Release of ^{13}C-Choline from rat bladder strips 5 days following injection with saline (sham) or 50 U onabotulinumtoxinA. Each value is the mean ± standard error of mean from 3 to 4 experiments. Note the significant decrease in release of acetylcholine from onabotulinumtoxinA treated rats at the higher frequency (20 Hz), $p<0.05$ (Copyright obtained from Smith et al. 2003a)

2.7.2 Afferent Effect

BoNT's efficacy in conditions of detrusor overactivity may result not only from an inhibitory effect on detrusor muscle, but some effects of the drug may be mediated by altering afferent (sensory) input. Urothelium possesses muscarinic receptor populations with a density two times as high as detrusor smooth muscle, and dorsal root ganglionectomy experiments demonstrating the persistence of acetylcholinesterase staining nerves near the urothelium suggest that parasympathetic nerves supply some innervation to urothelium (Hawthorn et al. 2000). Besides receiving cholinergic innervation, human urothelium, has also been shown to release the neurotransmitter acetylcholine at rest (Andersson and Yoshida 2003). Acetylcholine released from urothelium and acting on nearby muscarinic receptor populations (i.e., urothelium or afferent nerves) or neuronal sources of acetylcholine binding to muscarinic receptors within urothelium or afferent nerves could have a significant impact on bladder sensory input to the central nervous system and may be impacted by BoNT treatment.

In addition, recent basic and clinical evidence suggests that BoNT may have sensory inhibitory effects unrelated to its actions on acetylcholine release. For example, an in vitro model of mechanoreceptor-stimulated urothelial ATP release was tested in spinal cord injured rat bladders to determine whether intravesical botulinum toxin A administration would inhibit urothelial ATP release, a measure of sensory nerve activation (Khera et al. 2004). The results demonstrated that hypoosmotic stimulation of bladder urothelium evoked a significant release of ATP that was markedly inhibited by BoNT. This suggests that impairment of urothelial ATP release may be one mechanism by which BoNT reduces detrusor overactivity. BoNT has also been shown to inhibit release of neuropeptides such as calcitonin generelated peptide, substances thought to play a role in overactive bladder conditions such as sensory urgency or chronic bladder inflammation (i.e., interstitial cystitis) (Rapp et al. 2006; Chuang et al. 2004).

2.7.3 Effects on Acetylcholine and ATP Release

In animal bladder models, BoNT inhibited the release of acetylcholine in response to high-grade stimulation, but not low-grade stimulation (Smith et al. 2003b) (Fig. 2.3), suggesting that it may act on the muscarinic facilitatory mechanism mediated by protein kinase C.

ATP has also been implicated as a neurotransmitter in the generation of unstable contractions in idiopathic detrusor overactivity (Bayliss et al. 1999; O'Reilly et al. 2002). Studies on guinea pig (MacKenzie et al. 1982) and rat (Smith et al. 2003a) bladder strips have shown that BoNT is capable of inhibiting the release of both acetylcholine and ATP, providing a rationale for its possible use in treating patients with idiopathic overactive bladder.

Bladder urothelium may play an important role in the sensory transduction mechanisms modulating micturition, particularly in conditions of increased sensory nerve transmission following chronic inflammation and spinal cord injury (Khera et al. 2004). Urothelial cells can release ATP (Birder et al. 2002), and the increased release of ATP from the urothelium of spinal cord injured rat bladders could activate purine $P2X_3$ receptors in epithelial and subepithelial layers to increase afferent nerve activity, accounting for the higher frequency of bladder contractions seen in both human and animal models of spinal cord injury.

Recently, BoNT was shown to inhibit ATP release from the urothelium but not the serosal side of the bladder, suggesting that BoNT treatment inhibits neurotransmitter release not only from efferent nerve endings but from sensory nerve terminals and/or urothelium as well (Khera et al. 2004). BoNT significantly impairs urothelial ATP release following spinal cord injury presents a plausible explanation for its clinical efficacy in the treatment of human neurogenic bladder dysfunction.

2.7.4 Effect on Hot and Cold Sensitive Sensory Receptors

Originally described as a capsaicin receptor related to natural irritants (called vanilloids), the Transient Receptor Potential channel Vanilloid family member 1 (TRPV1) receptor is believed to function as an integrator of noxious stimuli, such as acids, heat, pollutants with a negative electronic charge, and endogenous pro-inflammatory substances. TRPV1 plays a key role in the perception of peripheral thermal and inflammatory pain (Morenilla-Palao et al. 2004). Recent findings indicate that BoNT blocks TRPV1 membrane translocation induced by protein kinase C, suggesting that activity-dependent delivery of channels to the neuronal surface may contribute to the buildup and maintenance of thermal inflammatory hyperalgesia in peripheral nociceptor terminals (Morenilla-Palao et al. 2004).

Successful BoNT treatment for overactive bladder is associated with a significant decrease of TRPV1 and/or $P2X_3$ in suburothelial nerve fibers (Apostolidis et al. 2005). These changes may reflect a direct effect of BoNT on the afferent innervation of the bladder and may occur as a secondary effect to the action of BoNT on the efferent innervation of the detrusor.

2.7.5 Clinical Effects on Calcitonin Gene-Related Peptide and Substance P Release

Sensory axons in the bladder contain both calcitonin gene-related peptide (CGRP) and substance P. These neuropeptides, which are released from nociceptive sensory endings in response to noxious stimuli, function as inflammatory response mediators (Basbaum and Jessell 2000). Substance P acts on mast cells to produce degranulation, resulting in release of histamine and cytokines, which directly sensitize or excite nociceptors. In addition, both substance P and CGRP produce edema (substance P through plasma extravasation, and CGRP through dilation of peripheral blood vessels), causing liberation of bradykinin, all of which can lead to further activation of primary afferent fibers (Basbaum and Jessell 2000). Together with bradykinin and prostaglandins, substance P and CGRP also cause migration of leukocytes to the site of injury and clotting responses (Aoki 2005; Zubrzycka and Janecka 2000).

BoNT has been shown in several preclinical models to block the release of CGRP, substance P, and glutamate from afferent nerve terminals (Aoki 2005; Chuang et al. 2004). The effect of BoNT on sensory pathways is supported by results reported in preclinical models of bladder pain, in which intravesical application of BoNT significantly reduced pain responses and inhibited CGRP release from afferent nerve terminals, suggesting that BoNT may have clinical applications for the treatment of disorders such as interstitial cystitis and sensory urgency (Chuang et al. 2004; Rapp et al. 2006).

2.7.6 Inhibition of Nerve Growth Factor Release and Receptor Transport

In both animals and humans, the bladder increases production of nerve growth factor (NGF) in response to conditions such as spinal cord injury, denervation, inflammation, distension, or hypertrophy (Steers and Tuttle 2006). NGF is a signaling protein that interacts with specific receptors along autocrine, paracrine and endocrine pathways. It is produced in the smooth muscle of the urinary tract and urothelium of the bladder, and elevated NGF levels have been reported to trigger bladder overactivity, such as that seen in men with benign prostatic hyperplasia, women with interstitial cystitis, and in patients with idiopathic overactive bladder.

Intravesical BoNT injection reduces nerve growth factor content in the bladder tissue of patients with neurogenic detrusor overactivity but it is unknown whether reduced bladder NGF results from decreased production, decreased uptake or a combination of both (Steers and Tuttle 2006). The result of this action of BoNT is to decrease the hyperexcitability of C-fiber bladder afferents, thereby reducing neurogenic detrusor overactivity (Giannantoni et al. 2006).

2.8 Histological Impact of BoNT Injection

Haferkamp et al. (2004) evaluated ultrastructural changes in overactive human detrusor tissue following BoNT injection in 30 biopsies from 24 patients with a diagnosis of neurogenic overactive bladder. Biopsies were taken before and 3 months after BoNT injection and during the wearing-off phase of the toxin's efficacy. They observed no significant changes in muscle cell fascicles, intercellular collagen content or muscle cell degeneration when comparing biopsies taken before and after BoNT administration, although these results cannot be extrapolated to the possible structural effects of repeat injections. Unlike striated muscle, axonal sprouting in detrusor smooth muscle was limited following BoNT administration, and further research is required to determine if prolonged toxin dosing will elicit such a response. The results of an immunohistochemical study also suggested no significant axonal sprouting in the suburothelium of successfully treated patients (Apostolidis et al. 2005).

A recent study reported histopathological changes in excised human neurogenic overactive bladders that could be associated with intradetrusor BoNT injections. Full-thickness specimens from bladders previously treated with one or more injections of BoNT showed significantly less fibrosis, but no differences in inflammation and edema compared to untreated ones; degrees of inflammation, edema and fibrosis were comparable in the two groups. Treated bladders had been injected with a mean number of 1.5 ± 0.8 injections, and the mean time between the last injection and surgery was 6.8 ± 2.8 months (Comperat et al. 2006).

Because the action of BoNT is reversible over time and does not appear to induce any enduring pathological changes, it has theoretical longevity in terms of its clinical usefulness in urological dysfunction. Indeed, regular BoNT blockade of striated muscle activity over a 12-year period was shown to be clinically safe and effective (Mejia et al. 2005). However, since biopsies were not performed, the long-term effects at a cellular level cannot be determined.

Although the majority of long-term results are positive, more data is needed from both smooth and striated muscle. A case study by Coletti Moja and colleagues has described acute neuromuscular failure in a patient who had a 2-year history of regular abobotulinumtoxinA treatment (800–1,000 U every 3 months for limb spasticity) (Coletti Moja et al. 2004). Biopsy investigations showed subacute denervation and inflammation of the deltoid muscle with unspecified diffuse abnormalities of group II afferent fibers at a site distal to the area of drug administration, with clinical features resembling an acute myasthenic-like syndrome. Such findings indicate that there is still much to learn about the effects of long-term exposure to BoNT.

2.9 BoNT Antibody Production

Questions remain about the long-term use of BoNT and the potential for development of resistance, with repeated treatments often leading to a progressive decline in therapeutic response. It has been suggested that this decline may be caused by development of neutralizing antibodies to BoNT. The functionally relevant antigenicity of a BoNT preparation depends upon the amount of botulinum toxin presented to the immune system, which is in turn determined by the specific biological activity and the relationship between the biological activity and the amount of botulinum neurotoxin contained in the preparation (Dressler and Hallett 2006).

It is important to remember that almost all of the published papers on the presence of antibodies have been based on use of the original onabotulinumtoxinA (Botox) formulation. The current formulation has a much lower protein load and a reduced incidence of antibody production. OnabotulinumtoxinA (Botox), AbobotulinumtoxinA (Dysport) and RimabotulinumtoxinB (Myobloc) specific biological activities are 60, 100, and 5 equivalent mouse U/ng neurotoxin, respectively (one mouse unit = the intraperitoneally administered dose that would be lethal for 50% of a group of 20 g mice). This translates into antibody-induced cervical dystonia failure rates of approximately 5%, 5%, and 44% for OnabotulinumtoxinA, AbobotulinumtoxinA and RimabotulinumtoxinB, respectively.

The results of recent long-term studies suggest that although resistance to BoNT is a clinical possibility, it is not a significant concern when considering the appropriate and safe use of the currently available formulations (with the possible exception of patients who may have had extended exposure to the original onabotulinumtoxinA formulation). It is important to note that if a patient does not respond to a particular injection, this does not necessarily indicate that the patient has developed blocking antibodies. In fact, the same patient may respond at a subsequent visit to exactly the same dose injected in the same muscles.

2.10 Conclusion

Botulinum toxin is efficacious across a wide variety of disorders that involve pathological neuromuscular activity. Advances have been made in our understanding of how BoNT works at a molecular level, yet questions remain. Further research is needed to characterize the protein receptors to which BoNT binds, to expand our understanding of light chain translocation within the motor neuron, to establish the process by which the light chain interacts with SNARE proteins, and to explore the toxin's long-term effects on smooth muscle cells.

Although there has been speculation that diffusion and proteolysis of the toxin's light chain eventually occurs, the mechanism that accounts for the durability as well as the loss of toxin action remains to be determined. Therapy with BoNT would appear to not only help alleviate muscle spasticity, but, in view of its proposed antinociceptive properties and impact on sensory feedback loops, could provide substantial relief of hyperalgesia associated with a variety of lower urinary tract disorders.

Box 2.1: Key Points of BoNT Mechanisms of Action
- There has been recent interest in the potential use of botulinum toxins, particularly onabotulinumtoxinA, in patients with detrusor overactivity and other urological disorders.
- After internalization of BoNT-A into the cytosol of presynaptic neurons, it disrupts fusion of the acetylcholine-containing vesicle with the neuronal wall by cleaving the SNAP-25 protein in the synaptic fusion complex.
- In detrusor overactivity, the effect of BoNT-A results in selective paralysis of the low-grade contractions of the unstable detrusor, while still allowing the high-grade contractions that initiate micturition.
- BoNT-A also seems to affect afferent nerve activity by modulating the release of ATP in the urothelium, blocking the release of substance P, calcitonin gene-related peptide and glutamate from afferent nerves, and reducing the levels of nerve growth factor.
- In view of its effects on sensory feedback loops, BoNT-A could have a potential role in relieving hyperalgesia associated with lower urinary tract disorders, in addition to its reported beneficial effects on symptoms of overactive bladder.

References

Andersson KE, Yoshida M (2003) Antimuscarinics and the overactive detrusor – which is the main mechanism of action. Eur Urol 43:1–5

Aoki KR (2005) Review of a proposed mechanism for the antinociceptive action of botulinum toxin type A. Neurotoxicology 26:785–793

Apostolidis A, Popat R, Yiangou Y et al (2005) Decreased sensory receptors P2X3 and TRPV1 in suburothelial nerve fibers following intradetrusor injections of botulinum toxin for human detrusor overactivity. J Urol 174:977–982

Ashton AC, Dolly JO (1988) Characterization of the inhibitory action of botulinum neurotoxin type A on the release of several transmitters from rat cerebrocortical synaptosomes. J Neurochem 50:1808–1816

Atiemo H, Wynes J, Chuo J, Nipkow L, Sklar GN, Chai TC (2005) Effect of botulinum toxin on detrusor overactivity induced by intravesical adenosine triphosphate and capsaicin in a rat model. Urology 65:622–626

Barinaga M (1993) Secrets of secretion revealed. Science 260:487

Basbaum AI, Jessell TM (2000) The perception of pain. In: Kandel ER, Schwartz JH, Jessell TM (eds) Principles of neural science, 4th edn. McGraw Hill, New York, pp 472–491

Bayliss M, Wu C, Newgreen D, Mundy AR, Fry CH (1999) A quantitative study of atropine-resistant contractile responses in human detrusor smooth muscle, from stable, unstable and obstructed bladders. J Urol 162:1833–1839

Birder LA, Nakamura Y, Kiss S et al (2002) Altered urinary bladder function in mice lacking the vanilloid receptor TRPV1. Nat Neurosci 5:856–860

Blasi J, Chapman ER, Link E et al (1993) Botulinum neurotoxin A selectively cleaves the synaptic protein SNAP-25. Nature 365:160–163

Chuang YC, Yoshimura N, Huang CC, Chiang PH, Chancellor MB (2004) Intravesical botulinum toxin A administration produces analgesia against acetic acid induced bladder pain responses in rats. J Urol 172:1529–1532

Coletti Moja M, Dimanico U, Mongini T, Cavaciocchi V, Gerbino Promis PC, Grasso E (2004) Acute neuromuscular failure related to long-term botulinum toxin therapy. Eur Neurol 51:181–183

Comperat E, Reitz A, Delcourt A, Capron F, Denys P, Chartier-Kastler E (2006) Histologic features in the urinary bladder wall affected from neurogenic overactivity – a comparison of inflammation, oedema and fibrosis with and without injection of botulinum toxin type A. Eur Urol 50:1058–1064

Cui M, Khanijou S, Rubino J, Aoki KR (2004) Subcutaneous administration of botulinum toxin A reduces formalin-induced pain. Pain 107:125–133

DasGupta BR (1994) Structures of botulinum neurotoxin, its functional domains, and perspectives on the crystalline type A toxin. In: Jankovic J, Hallett M (eds) Therapy with botulinum toxin. Marcel Dekker, New York, pp 15–39

Datta SN, Roosen A, Pullen A, Popat R, Rosenbaum TP, Elneil S, Dasqupta P, Fowler CJ, Apostolidis A (2010) Immunohistochemical expression of muscarinic receptors in the urothelium and suburothelium of neurogenic and idiopathic overactive human bladders, and changes with botulinum neurotoxin administration. J Urol 184:2578–2585

Dong M, Yeh F, Tepp WH, Dean C, Johnson EA, Janz R, Chapman ER (2006) SV2 is the protein receptor for botulinum neurotoxin A. Science 312(5773):592–596

Dolly JO, Black J, Williams RS, Melling J (1984) Acceptors for botulinum neurotoxin reside on motor nerve terminals and mediate its internalization. Nature 307:457–460

Dressler D, Hallett M (2006) Immunological aspects of Botox, Dysport, and Myobloc/NeuroBloc. Eur J Neurol 13(Suppl 1):11–15

Giannantoni A, Di Stasi SM, Nardicchi V et al (2006) Botulinum-A toxin injections into the detrusor muscle decrease nerve growth factor bladder tissue levels in patients with neurogenic detrusor overactivity. J Urol 175:2341–2344

Gilio F, Curra A, Lorenzano C, Modugno N, Manfredi M, Berardelli A (2000) Effects of botulinum toxin type A on intracortical inhibition in patients with dystonia. Ann Neurol 48:20–26

Haferkamp A, Schurch B, Reitz A, Krengel U, Grosse J, Kramer G, Schumacher S, Bastian PJ, Buttner R, Muller SC, Stohrer M (2004) Lack of ultrastructural detrusor changes following endoscopic injection of botulinum toxin type A in overactive neurogenic bladder. Eur Urol 46:784–791

Hawthorn MH, Chapple CR, Cock M, Chess-Williams R (2000) Urothelium-derived inhibitory factor(s) influence detrusor muscle contractility in vitro. Br J Pharmacol 129:416–419

Khera M, Somogyi GT, Kiss S, Boone TB, Smith CP (2004) Botulinum toxin A inhibits ATP release from bladder urothelium after chronic spinal cord injury. Neurochem Int 45:987–993

MacKenzie I, Burnstock G, Dolly JO (1982) The effects of purified botulinum neurotoxin type A on cholinergic, adrenergic and non-adrenergic, atropine-resistant autonomic neuromuscular transmission. Neuroscience 7:997–1006

Mejia NI, Vuong KD, Jankovic J (2005) Long-term botulinum toxin efficacy, safety, and immunogenicity. Mov Disord 20:592–597

Morenilla-Palao C, Planells-Cases R, Garcia-Sanz N, Ferrer-Montiel A (2004) Regulated exocytosis contributes to protein kinase C potentiation of vanilloid receptor activity. J Biol Chem 279:25665–25672

O'Reilly BA, Kosaka AH, Knight GF, Chang TK, Ford AP, Rymer JM, Popert R, Burnstock G, McMahon SB (2002) P2X receptors and their role in female idiopathic detrusor instability. J Urol 167:157–164

Rapp DE, Turk KW, Bales GT, Cook SP (2006) Botulinum toxin type a inhibits calcitonin gene-related peptide release from isolated rat bladder. J Urol 175:1138–1142

Schiavo G, Rossetto O, Santucci A et al (1992) Botulinum neurotoxins are zinc proteins. J Biol Chem 267:23479

Schiavo G, Santucci A, Dasgupta BR, Mehta PP, Jontes J, Benfenati F, Wilson MC, Montecucco C (1993) Botulinum neurotoxins serotypes A and E cleave SNAP-25 at distinct COOH-terminal peptide bonds. FEBS Lett 335:99–103

Schurch B, de Seze M, Denys P et al (2005) Botulinum toxin type a is a safe and effective treatment for neurogenic urinary incontinence: results of a single treatment, randomized, placebo controlled 6-month study. J Urol 174:196–200

Smith CP, Chancellor MB (2004) Emerging role of botulinum toxin in the management of voiding dysfunction. J Urol 171(6 Pt 1):2128–2137

Smith CP, Franks ME, McNeil BK, Ghosh R, de Groat WC, Chancellor MB, Somogyi GT (2003a) Effect of botulinum toxin A on the autonomic nervous system of the rat lower urinary tract. J Urol 169(5):1896

Smith CP, Boone TB, de Groat WC, Chancellor MB, Somogyi GT (2003b) Effect of stimulation intensity and botulinum toxin isoform on rat bladder strip contractions. Brain Res Bull 61:165

Steers WD, Tuttle JB (2006) Mechanisms of disease: the role of nerve growth factor in the pathophysiology of bladder disorders. Nat Clin Pract Urol 3:101–110

Zubrzycka M, Janecka A (2000) Substance P: transmitter of nociception (minireview). Endocr Regul 34:195–201

Part II
Bladder

Botulinum Toxin for Neurogenic Detrusor Overactivity

3.1 Introduction

Patients with neurogenic bladder dysfunction suffer from detrusor overactivity (detrusor hyperreflexia), which may be combined with detrusor sphincter dyssynergia (DSD; uncoordinated voiding). Both conditions cause high intravesical pressure and can lead to upper urinary tract damage.

Normal micturition is based on synergy between a functional bladder and a competent urethral sphincter. The bladder must function to store and empty urine properly, and the neural control resides in the pons and the suprapontine regions of the brain stem to switch between these two modes efficiently and appropriately. Neurogenic detrusor overactivity (NDO) occurs in upper motor neuron diseases or injury with lesions above the sacral spinal cord bladder micturition center. For those with spinal cord lesions, DSD or uncoordinated micturition between the bladder and sphincter may occur (Fig. 3.1). This conditions can cause high intravesical pressure and can lead to upper urinary tract damage.

Treatment for both DSD and detrusor overactivity can include pharmacologic therapy, catheterization, and surgery. Currently available pharmacologic treatments are often insufficient or not well tolerated.

3.2 Indications

It should be remembered that the majority of data on botulinum toxin injection for neurogenic detrusor overactivity are from the two groups of NDO patients, spinal cord injury, and multiple sclerosis, included in the registry trials for regulatory approval. Table 3.1 lists some of the neurological conditions that can cause neurogenic bladder dysfunction and where botulinum toxin may be considered as a treatment option.

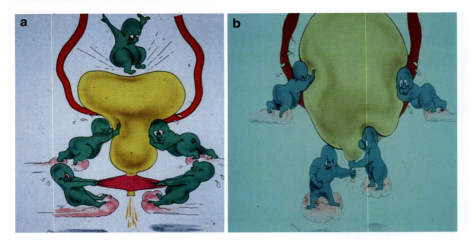

Fig. 3.1 Cartoon illustration of the two manifestations of neurogenic bladder dysfunction with overactive bladder. (**a**) Neurogenic detrusor overactivity with involuntary detrusor contractions but with synergistic sphincter and (**b**) neurogenic detrusor overactivity with detrusor-sphincter dyssynergia

Table 3.1 Neurological conditions frequently associated with neurogenic detrusor overactivity

Spinal cord conditions (with or without detrusor sphincter dyssynergia)
- Spinal cord injury
- Multiple sclerosis
- Transverse myelitis
- Tropical spastic paraparesis
- Myelomeningocele
- Tethered cord syndrome and short filum terminale
- Ankylosing spondylosis and disc disease
- Acquired immune deficiency syndrome

Supraspinal conditions (without detrusor sphincter dyssynergia)
- Cerebrovascular accident
- Cerebral palsy
- Parkinson's disease
- Dementia
- Neoplasm
- Cerebellar ataxia

3.2.1 Spinal Cord Injury

Approximately 10,000 spinal cord injuries (SCI) occur each year, most of which occur in males (80%). The US Model SCI Center maintains excellent data (http://www.spinalcord.uab.edu/show.asp?durki=19679). A majority of SCI patients suffer from bladder dysfunction and a combination of NDO with and without DSD can lead to long-term complications in up to 50% of patients (Kaplan et al. 1991;

3.2 Indications

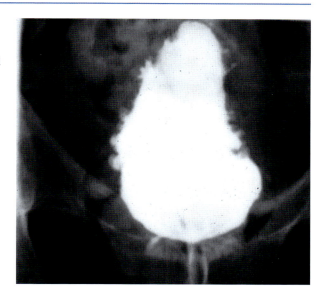

Fig. 3.2 Cystogram illustrating severe bladder trabeculation, a common finding in spinal cord injured patients with neurogenic detrusor overactivity. The shape and thickness of the neurogenic bladder dysfunction is often referred to as a Christmas or pine tree bladder

Woodside and McGuire 1979; Yalla et al. 1977). These complications include hydronephrosis, autonomic dysreflexia, vesicoureteral reflux, nephrolithiasis, sepsis, renal insufficiency or failure and even death. Figure 3.2 is a cystogram illustrating the severe trabeculation seen in SCI patients with neurogenic detrusor overactivity. The shape and thickness of the neurogenic bladder dysfunction is often referred to as a Christmas or pine tree or pine tree bladder. SCI patients often suffer from urinary incontinence which can lead to adverse events such as urinary tract infections and decubitus ulcers in addition to creating a large care burden for family members or healthcare providers and significantly impairing patient quality of life. Bladder problems related to SCI have a negative impact not only on a patient's physical condition, but also on their emotional and social well-being.

3.2.2 Multiple Sclerosis: Variable Spectrum and Disease Progression

Multiple sclerosis (MS) patients with neurogenic detrusor overactivity and detrusor sphincter dyssynergia needing intermittent self catheterization have similar characteristics and similar treatment guidance as SCI patients. But one should keep in mind that MS affects more women than men with a variable spectrum of disease severity that waxes and wanes. The disease is insidious in onset, often changes over time with disease progression that is characterized by relapses and yet long periods of stability. A key management issue is that many MS patients with milder manifestations of neurogenic bladder have NDO but do not have associated outlet obstruction related to DSD, so do not need to self-catheterize. Moreover, because of muscle weakness and spasticity, many MS patients lack the dexterity to perform intermittent self catheterization even if the ultimate goal of therapy is to completely paralyze the bladder. This is a critical management issue before considering bladder BoNT injection. The amount of BoNT and technique of injection may need to be modified, with a lower dose considered to help the MS patient achieve continence without retention or a significantly increased residual urine volume that would necessitate catheterization.

3.2.3 Pediatric Neurogenic Bladders

Children with NDO, especially those with myelodysplasia and cerebral palsy are potential candidates for bladder BoNT therapy. There are several studies in pediatric NDO demonstrating the safety and efficacy of BoNT. However, pediatric NDO was not included in international registry trials. We will discuss urologic applications of botulinum toxin use in children separately in Chap. 6.

3.2.4 Parkinson's Disease and Multisystem Atrophy

Lower urinary tract symptoms such as frequency, urgency, and urge incontinence are commonly found in patients suffering from Parkinson's disease, with prevalence rates between 27% and 40% (Fowler 2007; Winge et al. 2006). Urinary symptoms are even more common in multiple system atrophy (45–95%), thought to be a more severe form of Parkinson's disease. Detrusor hyperactivity is thought to result from a loss of dopaminergic-mediated tonic inhibition of micturition. Giannantoni and colleagues evaluated the effect of bladder injection with BoNT in six patients suffering from either Parkinson's disease (four patients) or multiple system atrophy (2 patients) (Giannantoni et al. 2009). One and three months after injection with 200 U onabotulinumtoxinA, all patients demonstrated significant reductions in frequency and nocturia and no further incontinence episodes were reported. The two patients with multiple system atrophy required intermittent catheterization. Parkinson's patients often display impaired urethral relaxation (i.e., sphincter bradykinesia) in addition to detrusor overactivity that theoretically could place them at risk for retention following onabotulinumtoxinA injection. Interestingly, none of the four Parkinson's disease patients required intermittent catheterization postoperatively. Larger studies are needed to determine the therapeutic role of BoNT in this subgroup of neurogenic bladder patients.

3.3 What Is the Work-Up?

3.3.1 History and Physical Examination

One should do a complete history including symptoms related to the neurologic injury or disease. Past medical history including medical and surgical history is required and response to any medications, especially if they have had BoNT in the past. Urogenital issues including sexual history, bladder diary, and fecal continence status should be addressed. Neurogenic functional status, ambulation status, and hand dexterity are of particular importance. Catheter usage and the ability to do catheterization is a high priority before considering BoNT. Home and social setting play a role in developing a realistic plan.

3.3.2 Urodynamic Evaluation

Urodynamic testing plays a pivotal role in evaluating patients with neurogenic bladder. This is a valuable tool to establish baseline bladder pressures and behavior that can be used for the diagnosis, prognosis, and management of their disease. Annual urodynamic studies are often recommended to assess disease process changes, especially in those with febrile infection, high bladder pressures, poor bladder compliance, or hydronephrosis or reflux. Urodynamic parameters recorded include: bladder sensation, filling pressure, capacity, compliance, uninhibited detrusor contractions, and residual volume. The sine qua non of neurogenic detrusor overactivity diagnosis is the presence of involuntary (i.e., uninhibited) detrusor contractions with bladder filling during urodynamic evaluation. Electromyography can be performed concurrently to diagnose DSD (Fig. 3.3). When combined with fluoroscopy, additional data on the mechanics, anatomy, and structure of the bladder, urethra, and the presence of vesicoureteral reflux can be obtained in real time. We have found video-urodynamics as the most reliable and detailed evaluation available prior to treating patients with neurogenic bladder.

3.4 How to Do It

3.4.1 Patient Preparation

Box 3.1 is an example of patient instruction sheet we give out to a patient prior to BoNT injection. Some key issues to consider are listed below. Procedures, guidelines, and rules may differ slightly among various centers and countries.
- Urine analysis should be negative at the time of the procedure (if the patient has a history of chronic bacteruria, appropriate preoperative antibiotic coverage is indicated).
- Anticoagulation medicine stopped for at least 5 days.
- Informed consent with notation of off-label use and drug warning.
- Sterile cystoscopic preparation with standard antibiotic coverage for a minor cystoscopic procedure.
- Latex allergy survey in this at risk population.
- In spinal cord injured patients with a history of autonomic dysreflexia or lesions above the T6 spinal cord level, precautions to deal with and procedures to minimize autonomic dysreflexia should be in place. Patient's blood pressure should be monitored and bladder overfilling should be avoided. Use of urethral and bladder local anesthesia is helpful and general anesthesia may need to be considered.

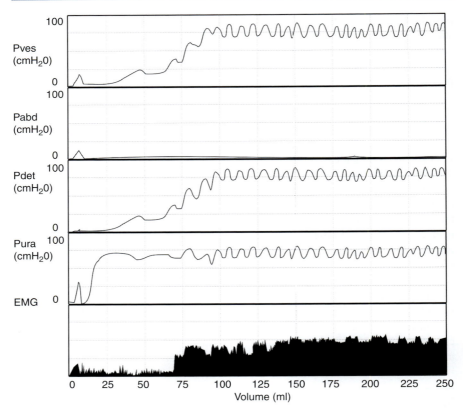

Fig. 3.3 Neurogenic detrusor overactivity with DSD: Note the elevated and sustained Pdet against a non-relaxing sphincter as noted by the increased EMG sphincter activity and high pressure in the membranous urethra (Pura) during involuntary detrusor contraction. *Pves* intravesical pressure, *Pabd* intraabdominal pressure, *Pura* intraurethral pressure at the level of the sphincter, *EMG* electromyography of the external sphincter. *Pdet* intradetrusor pressure: Pves – Pabd (cmH_2O)

Box 3.1: Patient Instruction for Botulinum Toxin Bladder Injection

The Day Before Treatment Session

NOTE: If you usually take oral antibiotics prior to dental appointments, we would like you to do the same before the bladder injection treatment session. Typically, such preventive antibiotic treatment is specifically given to patients with heart murmurs, mitral valve prolapse, and/or artificial joint replacements.

NOTE: Please remember that you may need to limit taking medications that affect bleeding prior to treatment. This includes aspirin, warfarin, and ibuprofen products. Please speak to us directly before the procedure about this. If you have taken such medicine please inform the nurse as soon as possible.

- As this is an office procedure performed solely with local anesthesia, it is not necessary for you to have someone drive you home.
- It is okay for you to eat and drink the morning of your treatment.

The Day of Treatment Session

NOTE: Please update your doctor about any new medications or other therapies. We would like to know about prescription medicines, over the counter medications, as well as any herbal/alternative remedies.

- The day of your study treatment, you will be asked to take a single dose of oral antibiotic to prevent a urine infection. Please bring a list of all your known medication allergies.
- Once you have been comfortably positioned on the procedure bed, the genital area will be sterilely washed and draped.
- A soft rubber catheter will be lubricated and inserted to drain the bladder empty of urine. Then before removing the same catheter, numbing liquid (1% lidocaine) will be pushed through the catheter into the bladder. No needles are used for this process to numb your bladder.
- After the numbing solution sits for 15 min, it will be drained and your doctor will proceed with the treatment.
- The cystoscope (camera type device) is guided into the bladder, allowing your doctor to inject the botulinum toxin medicine into the bladder wall. This injection process will take approximately 15 min to complete.
- After the treatment is finished, you will be asked to remain in the clinic for at least 30 min for observation. Also, we will ask that you urinate before leaving the office.
- If you are unable to satisfactorily urinate to empty your bladder (urinary retention), your doctor may want you to use a temporary catheter to drain the bladder.
- If your procedure is being done in the operating room as other procedures are also necessary, please note you will receive some sedation prior to examination and treatment.

What to Expect After Treatment

- You may notice some pain in your pelvic and and/or bladder area; some blood-tinged urine, as well as possible difficulty urinating. These symptoms should resolve within 24 h. Otherwise, please inform your doctor's office.
- The botulinum toxin medication will not work instantly. It may take several days or weeks to notice a gradual improvement in overactive bladder symptoms.

Risks of Treatment

Potential risks include bleeding, infection, and urinary retention. If urinary retention occurs, meaning you cannot empty your bladder, you may need to begin self-catheterization. This requires that you would place a tiny soft tube into your bladder several times per day to empty your bladder as it has become too relaxed to empty on its own.

> In addition, all botulinum toxin formulations must contain a Black Box Warning mandated by the FDA. Here is the Black Box Warning for onabotulinumtoxinA (Botox®, Allergan, Inc., Irvine, CA):
>
> BOTOX® and BOTOX® Cosmetic may cause serious side effects that can be life threatening. Call your doctor or get medical help right away if you have any of these problems after treatment with BOTOX® or BOTOX® Cosmetic:
> - Problems swallowing, speaking, or breathing. These problems can happen hours to weeks after an injection of BOTOX® or BOTOX® Cosmetic usually because the muscles that you use to breathe and swallow can become weak after the injection. Death can happen as a complication if you have severe problems with swallowing or breathing after treatment with BOTOX® or BOTOX® Cosmetic.
> - Swallowing problems may last for several months. People who already have swallowing or breathing problems before receiving BOTOX® or BOTOX® Cosmetic have the highest risk of getting these problems.
> - Spread of toxin effects. In some cases, the effect of botulinum toxin may affect areas of the body away from the injection site and cause symptoms of a serious condition called botulism. The symptoms of botulism include: loss of strength and muscle weakness all over the body, double vision, blurred vision and drooping eyelids, hoarseness or change or loss of voice (dysphonia), trouble saying words clearly (dysarthria), loss of bladder control, trouble breathing, trouble swallowing.

3.4.2 Cystoscope

Both rigid and flexible cystoscopic techniques work well in our hands and those of most experts without an apparent difference in clinical outcomes. Surgeon preference and institutional practice usually decide what technique should be used.

3.4.2.1 Rigid Cystoscope

While any rigid cystoscope will work, one author (CPS) prefers using an ACMI® Cystoscope with 12° lens, bridged with an Accessory Working Element loaded with a 25 gauge Cook® Williams Needle. The rigid scope allows for easier orientation within the bladder compared to a flexible cystoscope, the working element facilitates rapid injection into the bladder, and the 25 gauge needle minimizes bleeding and potential backflow from the injection sites.

The bladder volume is typically kept at 150–200 ml and blood vessels are avoided during injection. The first observable change is in urgency, frequency, and incontinence after 4–7 days, and all variables improve significantly after 4 weeks (Kalsi et al. 2008).

3.4.2.2 Flexible Cystoscope

We use flexible cystoscopy in the office for the majority of cases to minimize cost to patients if they are paying for the procedure out of pocket. The flexible scope

3.4 How to Do It

Fig. 3.4 (**a**) Close-up of the disposable injection needle (27 Fr, Olympus®) passed through a flexible cystoscope. (**b**) Cystogram image of flexible cystoscope inside a severely trabeculated bladder

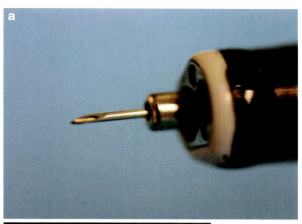

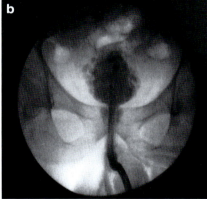

accommodates a 27 Fr flexible Olympus® injection needle (disposable) which must be passed through a reusable sheath (Fig. 3.4). Office procedures with only local anesthesia are adequate for most of our patients. Patients appreciate the convenience of an office procedure.

3.4.3 Botulinum Toxin Reconstitution

Each vial of 100 U onabotulinumtoxinA (Botox®, Allergan Inc., Irvine, CA) is usually reconstituted to 10 ml with injectable preservative-free saline, making the concentration equivalent to 10 U/ml. OnabotulinumtoxinA is kept in the refrigerator according to instruction and we usually do not reconstitute the onabotulinumtoxinA until we know that infection has been ruled out or an appropriate antibiotic started to avoid wastage.

Each vial of abobotulinumtoxinA (Dysport®, Ipsen Biopharm Ltd, Brisbane, CA) contains either 300 U (i.e., for Glabellar lines) or 500 U (i.e., for Cervical

Dystonia). Studies have documented dilutions with preservative-free saline to a concentration of 25–100 U/ml.

Each vial of rimabotulinumtoxinB (Myobloc®, US WorldMeds. Louisville, KY) contains 5,000 U/ml and, as opposed to onabotulinumtoxinA (i.e., vacuum-dried) and abobotulinumtoxinA (i.e., freeze-dried) preparations, is already reconstituted. Although few studies have used rimabotulinumtoxinB to treat bladder overactivity, most have diluted to a concentration of 250 U/ml.

3.4.4 Dose

We routinely use 200 U of onabotulinumtoxinA for first time injection in the majority of our NDO patients. We will use 100 U of onabotulinumtoxinA for our multiple sclerosis with NDO but who are not on self catheterization and would prefer not having to self catheterize if possible. Based on our experience, if the results are suboptimal we will increase the bladder injection dosage to 300 U and rarely 400 U in selective cases before considering augmentation. In cases of impaired muscle contraction/respiration, we lower our starting dose of onabotulinumtoxinA to 100 U. For pediatric patients, we generally start with a 100 U dose of onabotulinumtoxinA, although others have described doses up to 12 U/kg, similar to doses given in other neurologically impaired pediatric populations (Schulte-Baukloh et al. 2002). Typical doses in adult patients treated with abobotulinumtoxinA range between 500 and 1,000 U, and for rimabotulinumtoxinB range between 2,500 and 15,000 U (i.e., 5,000 U most common).

Box 3.2: Important Safety Warning

- The potency units of all commercially available botulinum toxins are specific to that particular preparation and assay method utilized.
- Different brands of botulinum toxins *are not* interchangeable with other preparations of botulinum toxin products.
- Therefore, units of biological activity of one toxin preparation cannot be compared or converted into units of any other botulinum toxins products assessed with any other specific assay method.

3.4.5 Depth, Location, and Amount of Injection

We usually inject 1 ml per site (10 U onabotulinumtoxinA/ml) so, for example, if we are using 200 U there will be approximately 20 injection sites. In this case we would take two bottles of 100 U of onabotulinumtoxinA and dissolve each bottle in 10 ml of preservative-free saline.

3.4.6 Injection Technique

How deep should BoNT be injected into the bladder? In a recent study using MRI for detecting the distribution of onabotulinumtoxinA throughout the bladder wall after injecting 300 U for NDO, 18% of the onabotulinumtoxinA solution was found outside the bladder dome and the remainder covered 25–33% of the bladder wall (Mehnert et al. 2009). In addition, Kuo demonstrated significant increases in functional bladder capacity and significant reductions in urge episodes without an increase in post-void residual in patients with idiopathic overactive bladder undergoing bladder trigone sub-urothelial injections compared to patients injected intramuscularly outside of the trigone (Kuo 2007). Without actually labeling onabotulinumtoxinA, one cannot be sure of how much of the bladder is covered with each injection paradigm. However, if beneficial effects are achieved with only 25–33% of the bladder wall covered, perhaps we are overtreating patients with a 30–40 injection template. Moreover, injection into the suburothelium might avoid the potential loss of BoNT through detrusor injections and allow for lower doses and more refined injection paradigms to be employed (Fig. 3.5).

Recent evidence in human cadaveric bladder tissues demonstrates that the BoNT-A receptor SV2 co-localizes with parasympathetic nerves within the suburothelium and detrusor muscle. Thus, both plexuses would be natural targets to deliver the toxin (Coelho et al. 2009). Recent studies of BoNT injection for idiopathic detrusor overactivity have used suburothelial delivery to potentially target the suburothelial sensory pathway rather than paralysis of detrusor muscle. However, in many NDO patients who are already catheterizing and where complete paralysis is the treatment objective, perhaps deeper detrusor injections should be the approach used. Unfortunately, especially in idiopathic detrusor overactive bladders with a thin bladder wall, it might be difficult to differentiate suburothelium from detrusor muscle.

3.4.6.1 Trigone Injection

A successful outcome was reported with BoNT injection into only the trigone and bladder base (Fig. 3.6) (Smith and Chancellor 2005). The rationale for trigone injection is that this portion of the urinary bladder contains a prominent parasympathetic plexus of BoNT-A receptor-positive nerves, although the role of this plexus on bladder urgency sensation and detrusor overactivity has not been fully explored (Coelho et al. 2009). This also does not take into account a possible therapeutic effect of BoNT on the abundant sensory nerves within the trigone.

Abdel-Meguid TA (2010) reported a prospective, randomized, controlled trial of trigonal injection in 36 patients. The patients were evenly randomized to either only detrusor injection excluding the trigone (300 U onabotulinumtoxinA) or intradetrusor (200 U onabotulinumtoxinA) plus intratrigonal injection (100 U onabotulinumtoxinA). Abdel-Meguid reported that all parameters improved significantly in each group with greater improvements in incontinence episodes, complete dry rate and larger duration of effect in the trigonal group. There were no new or worsened vesicoureteral reflux in either group.

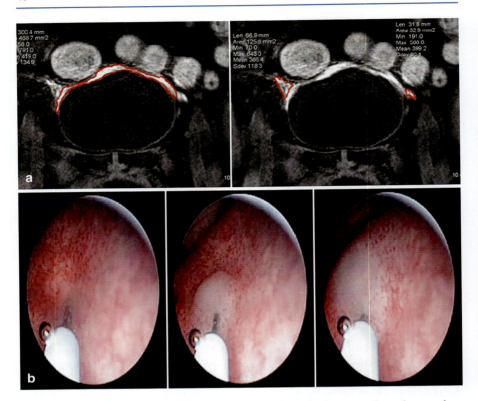

Fig. 3.5 Questions arise regarding how deep to inject the toxin: intramuscular, submucosal, or epithelial. (**a**) Mehnert and colleagues performed a study where NDO patient's bladders were injected intramuscularly with 300 U of onabotulinumtoxinA mixed with gadolinium (Copyright obtained, Mehnert et al. 2009) Immediately following injection, patients underwent an MRI study to document the distribution of the gadolinium. The investigators found that almost 18% of injected onabotulinumtoxinA was localized outside the bladder wall in the extraperitoneal fat. Our goal with bladder injections is to minimize the number of injections required by maximizing spread while preventing migration of the toxin into the retroperitoneal space. (**b**) The *middle panel* shows what we would consider "poor" injection technique. The needle placement is too shallow creating a blistering effect of the urothelium with loss of vascular markings and minimal toxin spread. As the needle is inserted further (i.e., *right panel*) the injection is then directed submucosally with significant elevation of the mucosal wall in both vertical and horizontal planes and persistence of mucosal vascular markings. We consider the *right panel* as "good" injection technique. In addition, because we have avoided intramuscular injection, our risk of extravesical extravasation is mitigated

Although vesicoureteral reflux might be a potential complication after BoNT in these areas, there is no evidence of it so far (Karsenty et al. 2007; Pinto et al. 2010; Smith et al. 2005). In the present authors' personal experience over the past 10 years, submucosal trigone and bladder base injections of BoNT are associated with a low incidence of urinary retention and a similar efficacy to intradetrusor injection.

3.4 How to Do It

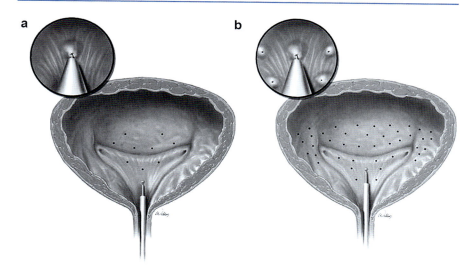

Fig. 3.6 Illustration depicting (**a**) modified 10-point BoNT injection technique within the bladder trigone and base we use in spontaneously voiding patients with mild to moderate overactive bladder symptoms and (**b**) traditional injection mapping of approximately 30–40 injection sites of BoNT within the trigone, bladder base and lateral walls that we use primarily to treat patients where complete bladder paralysis is the goal (Copyright obtained, Smith and Chancellor 2004)

It should be emphasized that no standardized injection technique exists for botulinum toxin injection in lower urinary tract tissues. Clinical success has been described using different bladder injection paradigms (i.e., trigone vs. trigone-sparing).

3.4.7 Simultaneous Bladder and Sphincter BoNT Injection

For select neurologically impaired patients with both NDO and DSD, injection of BoNT into the bladder and sphincter may be considered at the same treatment session.

3.4.7.1 Bladder Injection
Bladder injections with BoNT can be done using either a rigid or flexible cystoscope, under local anesthesia. A total of 100–200 U of onabotulinumtoxinA diluted in 10–20 ml of preservative free saline (i.e., 10 U/ml) are injected submucosally throughout the bladder using an endoscopic injection needle.

3.4.7.2 Sphincter Injection
One Hundred units of onabotulinumtoxinA are generally utilized in women and 200 U in men. Each 100 unit vial of onabotulinumtoxinA is diluted in 2 ml of preservative-free saline. For women, a 22 gauge short spinal needle is inserted

periurethrally for 1.5–2.0 cm at the 3 o'clock and 9 o'clock positions and 1 ml of onabotulinumtoxinA is injected at each site. Male urethral sphincters are injected with a total of 200 U of onabotulinumtoxinA diluted in 2 ml of preservative-free saline under local or general anesthesia with a rigid cystoscope using an endoscopic injection needle (e.g., 25 gauge Cook® Williams Needle). BoNT is injected in equal aliquots of 0.5 ml at the 12, 3, 6, and 9 o'clock positions. It is recommended that the injection be directed deeper than urethral bulking agent injection to target nerve terminals innervating the external (skeletal muscle) urethral sphincter.

Clinicians must make contingency plans after combined bladder/sphincter injection due to the fact that the duration of effect is longer following bladder injection (i.e., 6–9 months) than following sphincter injection (i.e., 3–4 months). This could include use of alpha blocker therapy or skeletal muscle relaxants (i.e., baclofen) to prolong the durability of sphincter injection until it is time to retreat the bladder.

3.4.8 Post-procedure and Follow-Up

We instruct our patients that they may notice some pain and blood-tinged urine, as well as possible difficulty urinating following treatment. These symptoms should resolve within 24 h and they should call and contact us immediately if they have any questions or concerns. We discuss the appropriate antibiotic coverage and risk of infection in these patients who often have more bladder infections. For those who are not already on intermittent catheterization, we formulate a plan if urinary retention occurs.

We reiterate that the botulinum toxin effect is not instantaneous. It may take several days to notice a gradual improvement in overactive bladder symptoms. Similarly, it generally takes several days for a patient to notice impaired voiding and we would instruct that patient to start self-catheterization if clinically necessary.

3.4.9 How Long Does It Last and When Is Botulinum Toxin Injection Repeated

It generally takes about 1 week for our patients to notice some relief of symptoms. If the injection helps, he or she will gain further improvement that usually reaches a maximal benefit at about 1 month. The beneficial effect is usually maintained for 6–9 months. Subsequently, urination or catheterization frequency starts to increase and incontinence reoccurs. These are signals we tell our patients to look for and to contact us to schedule a repeat injection.

3.4.10 Subsequent Dose Selection (Can You and Should You Go Up or Down on Dose)

For the majority of patients who notice a benefit with bladder BoNT therapy, we use the same dose with repeat injections. Most neurologically impaired patients have had consistent improvement using the same dose and frequency for over 10 years. If the patient finds benefit but incontinence did not completely resolve with 200 U onabotulinumtoxinA, we will consider going up to 300 U onabotulinumtoxinA with the next injection. In rare cases, such as spinal cord injured patients with long-term severe neurogenic bladder dysfunction, we have moved up to 400 U onabotulinumtoxinA, after determining that 300 U onabotulinumtoxinA is not enough.

Alternatively, in multiple sclerosis patients who do not perform self-catheterization but have noticed retention or incomplete bladder emptying, we generally start at 100 U onabotulinumtoxinA. If patients have previous received 200 U onabotulinumtoxinA but notice more difficulty with bladder emptying we will decrease the dose from 200 to 100 U onabotulinumtoxinA on subsequent treatments.

3.4.11 Risk of Antibody Formation

Failure to respond to BoNT injection might result from the presence of pre-existing BoNT antibodies (BoNT-AB; primary failure) or to the production of BoNT-AB's in response to BoNT injection (secondary failure). Neurologic literature has documented a sharp reduction in the incidence of onabotulinumtoxinA antibody formation from 9.5% to 0.5% in cervical dystonia patients with the introduction of a newer formulation of onabotulinumtoxinA in 1998 (i.e., reduced protein load from 25 ng/100 U to 5 ng/100 U) (Jankovic et al. 2003; Schulte-Baukloh et al. 2008). However, although BoNT use in urologic conditions has increased, little data exists on the risk of BoNT-AB formation in this patient population.

Schulte-Baukloh and colleagues determined the presence of onabotulinumtoxinA-ABs in patients treated multiple times with onabotulinumtoxinA and correlated the presence of antibodies with clinical response (Schulte-Baukloh et al. 2008). Eight of twenty-five patients had either elevated (four patients) or borderline elevated (four patients) onabotulinumtoxinA-AB serum titers. Interestingly, the authors found no correlation between the presence of onabotulinumtoxinA-ABs and the number of injections, time between injections, or total dose given. Three of five complete treatment failure patients had definitively elevated onabotulinumtoxinA-AB's and no other obvious reason for lack of response to repeated injection with onabotulinumtoxinA. The other two complete treatment failure patients without elevated onabotulinumtoxinA-ABs had obvious reasons for not responding to botulinum toxin treatment (i.e., poor compliance and tethered cord, respectively). The author's concluded that BoNT-AB formation appears to be more prevalent after botulinum toxin application to the bladder compared to skeletal muscle. They recommended a "drug holiday" in clinical non-responders with elevated BoNT-AB titers, as BoNT-ABs disappeared in two patients with borderline levels after 6 and 12 months, respectively.

3.5 What Are the Results

3.5.1 Clinical Studies

The use of onabotulinumtoxinA in the urinary bladder was first described in manuscript form by Schurch and colleagues who demonstrated a significant increase in mean maximum bladder capacity (296–480 ml, $p<0.016$) and a significant decrease in mean maximum detrusor voiding pressure (65–35 cmH$_2$O, $p<0.016$) in 21 patients with NDO that were injected with onabotulinumtoxinA (Schurch et al. 2000). Seventeen of nineteen patients were completely continent at 6 week follow-up, and were very satisfied with the procedure. Interestingly, baseline improvement in urodynamic parameters and incontinence persisted at 36-weeks in their follow-up of 11 patients. In the largest clinical series presented to date, a multicenter retrospective study examined 200 patients with neurogenic bladder treated with intravesical onabotulinumtoxinA injections (Del Popolo et al. 2008). At both 3- and 6-month follow-up, mean cystometric bladder capacity and mean voiding pressures decreased significantly.

Schurch and associates reported the first randomized, placebo-controlled trial examining the effects of two doses of onabotulinumtoxinA (i.e., 200 or 300 U) versus saline injection on various parameters including urodynamic measurements and urinary incontinence episodes (Schurch et al. 2005). Significant decreases in incontinent episodes (i.e., approximately 50%), significant increases in maximal cystometric capacity (i.e., approximately 170–215 ml), and significant improvements in quality of life scores were demonstrated in both onabotulinumtoxinA treatment groups compared to controls (Figs. 3.7–3.9). Beneficial effects lasted the duration of the study (i.e., 6 months). The study was not powered to detect statistical differences between the two onabotulinumtoxinA doses injected. Importantly, no safety concerns related to adverse events from onabotulinumtoxinA treatment were reported.

A second randomized, placebo-controlled trial compared the effect of abobotulinumtoxinA (500 units) versus placebo in patients with NDO. A total of 31 patients were treated (i.e., 17 with abobotulinumtoxinA and 14 with placebo) and 27 patients were available for follow-up (i.e., 17 abobotulinumtoxinA and 10 placebo) (Ehren et al. 2007). Similar increases in bladder capacity and similar reductions in maximum detrusor pressures were observed in the abobotulinumtoxinA randomized trial as compared to the onabotulinumtoxinA randomized trial. In addition, Ehren and colleagues noted significant improvement in quality of life and marked reduction in the amount of anticholinergic medication taken in patients treated with abobotulinumtoxinA. No safety concerns were raised in the abobotulinumtoxinA treated population.

3.5 What Are the Results

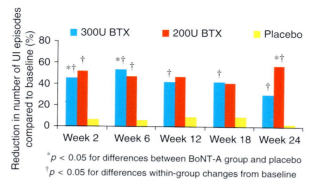

Fig. 3.7 Fifty nine patients with NDO underwent bladder injection with either: placebo, onabotulinumtoxinA 200 U, or onabotulinumtoxinA 300 U (Adapted from Schurch et al. 2005). Significant decreases in the number of incontinence episodes were documented in both onabotulinumtoxinA treatment groups at all time points except weeks 12 and 18 in the 200 U group. No placebo effect was demonstrated. Both treatment groups reduced incontinence episodes by approximately 50% compared to baseline

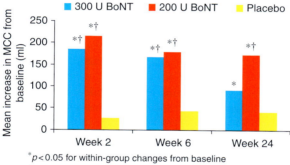

Fig. 3.8 Mean changes in maximal cystometric capacity were significantly higher in both onabotulinumtoxinA treatment groups compared to placebo at every time point except at week 24 in the 300 U onabotulinumtoxinA group (Adapted from Schurch et al. 2005). Mean increases in bladder capacity ranged from approximately 170–220 ml. No significant change in capacity was observed in the placebo group

One small randomized study evaluated the effect of rimabotulinumtoxinB compared to placebo in a mixed population of 20 patients with either neurogenic or non-neurogenic detrusor overactivity (Ghei et al. 2005). The study found significant improvements in voided volume, urinary frequency, incontinence episodes, and quality of life parameters in the rimaBoNT-B group compared to placebo. Unfortunately, subjects were followed for only 6 weeks and then crossed over to the other treatment paradigm, making it hard to clearly define the durability of effect.

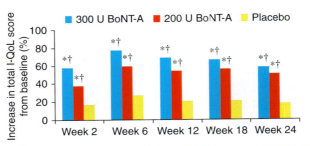

Fig. 3.9 Improvements in quality of life scores were noted (i.e., I-QOL) in both onabotulinumtoxinA treatment groups compared to placebo (Adapted from Schurch et al. 2005). Interestingly, the increased scores were maintained for the duration of the study (i.e., 24 weeks)

These randomized studies show that BoNT is more effective than placebo for improving the symptoms and signs of NDO, measured by the reduction in episodes of urinary incontinence as well as improvements in urodynamic parameters. BoNT serotype A has an acceptable safety profile when injected into the detrusor of patients with NDO. We have observed a sustained duration of efficacy of 6–9 months per injection and maintenance of efficacy with repeated injection of onabotulinumtoxinA of up to 10 years, with no clinical intolerance, or loss of efficacy due to antibody formation (Chancellor 2010).

What can one expect from injecting a NDO bladder with BoNT? Karsenty and colleagues summarized results of bladder injections with BoNT in NDO patients (Karsenty et al. 2008). Over 1,000 NDO patients have been examined in 25 studies detailing the effects of bladder BoNT injections. While significant variability in results were displayed if we summarize the findings of the five largest studies (i.e., all containing >50 patients) the following conclusions can be reached:

1. 73–95% of patients achieve complete continence
2. The frequency of patient leakage episodes is reduced by 32–90%
3. Mean cystometric capacity is increased by 40–178%
4. Maximal detrusor pressure is reduced by 22–51%

The results of Phase III clinical trials of OnaboutlinumtoxinA for NDO were recently reported by Ginsberg et al. (2011) and Chancellor et al., (2011). In an international multicenter, double-blind, randomized, placebo-controlled, parallel-group study, MS and SCI patients with urinary incontinence and NDO not adequately managed with anticholinergics were treated with intradetrusor onabotulinumtoxinA (200 or 300 U) or placebo. Patients were followed for up to 64 weeks and could request retreatment once from week 12 onward. The primary endpoint was the change from baseline in weekly UI episodes at week 6. Secondary endpoints included changes from baseline in urodynamic parameters and quality of life scores. The results reported patients of a mean age 46 years old with 30.5 weekly urinary incontinence episodes at baseline. The three treatment groups included placebo (*n*=149) onaBoNT-A 200 U (*n*=135), or onaBoNT-A 300 U (*n*=132). There were no significant differences between groups in baseline characteristics or urodynamics. The two studies noted significant and similar improvements in incontinence episodes; urodynamic parameters and health related quality of life scores with both 200 and 300 U onabotulinumtoxinA. Both doses were well tolerated.

3.5.2 Duration of Effect

The varying periods that each toxin effectively inhibits exocytosis depends on the differences in SNARE-binding profiles between the BoNT serotypes. BoNT-A, when used clinically for the treatment of dystonia, has by far the longest duration of activity, inducing clinical effects on neuromuscular activity for greater than 4 months, compared with a duration of effect of 2 months for BoNT-B or less than 4 weeks for BoNT-E (Eleopra et al. 1998; Sloop et al. 1997). Recovery of neurotransmission depends on the removal of the BoNT protease as well as the restoration of intact SNARE proteins (Foran et al. 2003; Keller and Neale 2001; Keller et al. 1999). In addition, structural differences in the end organs will lead to different duration of effects even with the same toxin. Mehnert and associates (2010) recently reported that in 12 patients with NDO due to multiple sclerosis treated with 100 U onabotulinumtoxinA clinical efficacy was achieved with a median time to re-injection of 8 months.

In general, most bladder studies document duration of effect of BoNT-A between 6 and 9 months. This has been our experience with our neurogenic and idiopathic OAB patients for over a decade.

3.5.3 Repeat Injections

3.5.3.1 OnabotulinumtoxinA and AbobotulinumtoxinA for NDO

Grosse and colleagues evaluated the effectiveness of repeated detrusor injections of onabotulinumtoxinA or abobotulinumtoxinA for NDO (Grosse et al. 2005). A total of 66 patients with refractory neurogenic detrusor overactivity received between 2 and 7 injections of onabotulinumtoxinA or abobotulinumtoxinA. The authors found significant and similar reductions in detrusor overactivity and in the use of anticholinergic medication in addition to significant increases in bladder capacity after injection one up to injection three (Fig. 3.10). The average interval between injections one and four was similar (i.e., approximately 9–11 months).

3.5.3.2 AbobotulinumtoxinA for NDO

The largest experience detailing the effect of abobotulinumtoxinA preparation on patients with NDO was described by Del Popolo and colleagues (Del Popolo et al. 2008). A total of 199 patients with NDO were treated over a 6 year period with 500, 750, or 1,000 IU of abobotulinumtoxinA. Significant improvements in urodynamic parameters (i.e., maximal bladder capacity, reflex volume) as well as significant reductions in incontinence episodes and pad usage were noted. Interestingly, median duration of effect did not differ between the three doses (12–13 months). Approximately 20% of patients responded for over 12 months. In addition, improvements in key urodynamic parameters were reproducible for up to seven injections.

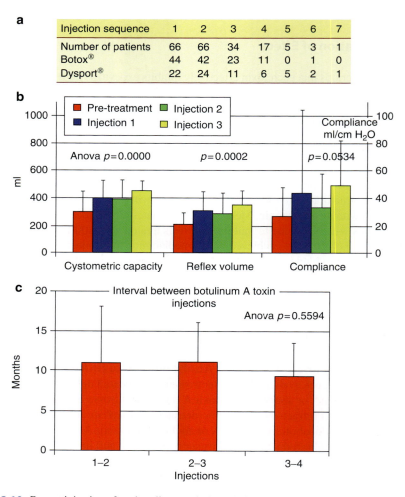

Fig. 3.10 Repeat injection of onabotulinumtoxinA or abobotulinumtoxinA for NDO. (Copyright obtained Grosse et al. 2005) (**a**) Grosse and colleagues evaluated the effectiveness of at least two detrusor injections in 42 patients treated with onabotulinumtoxinA and 24 patients treated with abobotulinumtoxinA. (**b**) Cystometric capacity and reflex volume improved significantly compared to baseline after injections 1–3. No significant change was noted in bladder compliance. (**c**) The interval between injections did not change between injection 1 and injection 4 (i.e., approximately 9–11 months) nor was a difference in interval observed between patients treated with onabotulinumtoxinA and abobotulinumtoxinA. (**d**) After the first injection, 31% of patients stopped anticholinergic medication use and 28% of patients decreased their dosage used. Significant decreases in anticholinergic medication use were maintained up to injection 3

3.5 What Are the Results

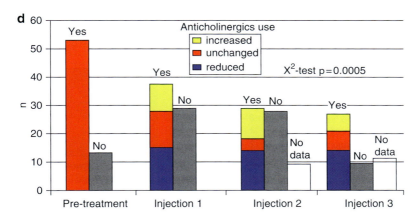

Fig. 3.10 (continued)

3.5.4 No Histological Damage to Bladder with BoNT Repeated Injections

Recent articles have examined the histological and ultrastructural effects of BoNT-A injection into the detrusor. While prior work in skeletal muscle demonstrated significant axonal sprouting following BoNT injection that eventually regressed (de Paiva et al. 1999), Haferkamp and colleagues found little evidence of axonal sprouting in bladder biopsies obtained from 24 patients with neurogenic detrusor overactivity following detrusor BoNT injection (Haferkamp et al. 2004). Understanding the differences in recovery of bladder parasympathetic versus somatic nerves may also provide a better insight into the mechanisms behind clinical differences in BoNT-A's duration of action. Not only does BoNT appear to have little effect on neuronal architecture within the bladder, but investigators have also shown that onabotulinumtoxinA does not induce bladder inflammation or edema (Comperat et al. 2006). Surprisingly, these same investigators found that patients treated with onabotulinumtoxinA displayed significantly less bladder wall fibrosis than non-treated patients. These findings should alleviate concerns of urologists that repeated detrusor injections with BoNT will induce bladder wall fibrosis and lead patients more rapidly to surgical options. It should also be of reassurance to patients who want BoNT to be a durable but reversible fix.

3.5.5 Can BoNT Improve Bladder Compliance?

While botulinum toxin has been shown to reduce detrusor overactivity in patients with neurogenic bladders, earlier studies did not investigate whether BoNT treatment could improve bladder compliance, and possibly, reduce the need for invasive surgery. Klaphajone and colleagues examined the effects of injecting 300 U of onabotulinumtoxinA into the detrusor muscle of ten spinal cord injured patients with

Fig. 3.11 Ten patients with documented poor bladder compliance underwent bladder injection with 300 U of onabotulinumtoxinA (Klaphajone et al. 2005). (**a**) Bladder compliance improved significantly from 6.5 ± 5.0 to 13.2 ± 5.2 ml/cmH$_2$O. (**b**) The mean volume at first reflex significantly increased from 54.1 ± 27.5 to 85.6 ± 27.4 ml. (**c**) Mean functional bladder capacity increased approximately 150 ml with treatment (i.e., 175.0 ± 56.2–331.1 ± 95.8 ml). (**d**) Maximal detrusor pressures decreased by over 50% well below 40 cmH$_2$O (60.4 ± 14.9–24.2 ± 10.2 cmH$_2$O). Urodynamic improvements were noted in all parameters at 6 and 16 weeks but became non-significant at 36 weeks follow-up

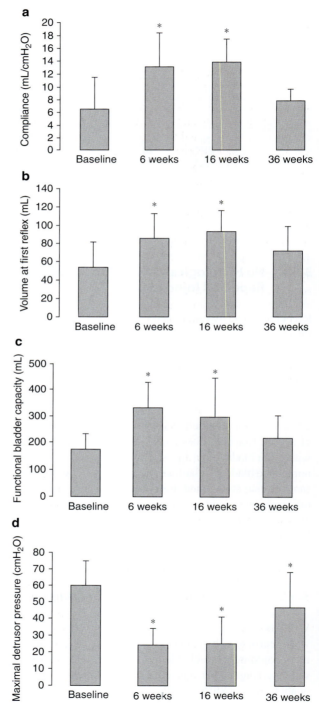

detrusor compliance ≤ 20 ml/cmH$_2$O (Klaphajone et al. 2005). Significant improvements were noted in mean bladder compliance (i.e., 6.5 ± 5.0 to 13.2 ± 5.2 ml/cmH$_2$O) and mean functional bladder capacity (i.e., mean increase of 156 ml) (Fig. 3.11). In addition, 70% of patients were completely continent at 6 weeks follow-up and continence was maintained in 50% of patients 9 months after injection. These results are in stark contrast to the poor results achieved in a separate study of eight patients with idiopathic bladder overactivity and poor detrusor compliance (Schmid et al. 2006). However, beneficial effects of BoNT in patients with poor detrusor compliance should only be expected if the decreased compliance is a result of increased neurogenic tone of the detrusor muscle and not secondary to bladder wall fibrosis. In addition, although the improvement in bladder compliance observed by Klaphajone and associates was significant, the post-treatment compliance remained poor at 13.2 ± 5.2 ml/cmH$_2$O. Many clinicians would be dissatisfied with the limited improvement in compliance observed by this study and would look at other alternatives (i.e., bladder augmentation). In this regard, these patients would be considered as having failed onabotulinumtoxinA treatment. One important question is, if and how, one can preoperatively predict whether a patient's poor compliance is related to increased fibrosis versus increased neuromuscular tone. In the latter case, patients should respond positively to BoNT injection. Perhaps a patient's response to antimuscarinic medication may give some insight into predicting if and by how much a patient's bladder compliance will improve after BoNT treatment.

> **Case 3.1: A 33-year-old spinal cord injury woman considering bladder augmentation**
> *Chief Complaint:* Incontinence between self-catheterization despite anticholinergics.
>   A 33-year-old spinal cord injury (SCI) woman on oxybutynin extended release 30 mg/day yet is incontinent and considering bladder augmentation. She suffered a (T-8) spinal cord injury after an auto accident. The patient works and finds the urine leakage between catheterization that she has to do every 2–3 years interfering with her life style. She has had leakage episodes during sex and she is not happy with fluid restriction which interferes with her social activities. The patient complains of dry mouth and constipation with her anticholinergics. The patient is engaged to be married and hesitant about bladder reconstruction and its affect on her appearance, bowel pattern, and future pregnancy risks (Fig. 3.12).
>   She decided to have onabotulinumtoxinA injection and understood it's off label use and potential risks. After informed consent, she underwent flexible cystoscopic injection of 200 U in 30 ml as an outpatient procedure under local anesthesia. At 2 month follow-up, the patient reported resolution of her leaking episodes and was able to stop her oxybutynin after 1 month. She also catheterizes her bladder six times a day compared to ten times a day before her procedure (Fig. 3.13). The efficacy was maintained for 6 months when she began noticing occasional leakage between catheterization and having to catheterize more often. She requested a repeat injection about a month before getting married.

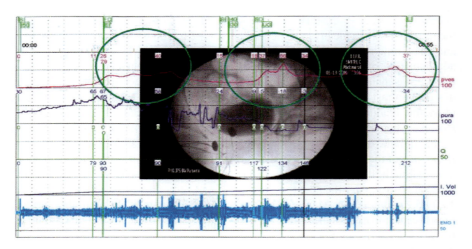

Fig. 3.12 Urodynamic tracing of a 33-year-old SCI woman on oxybutynin extended release 30 mg/day with leaking. Note the high pressure uninhibited contractions (i.e., *circled*) observed while on maximum dose antimuscarinic therapy

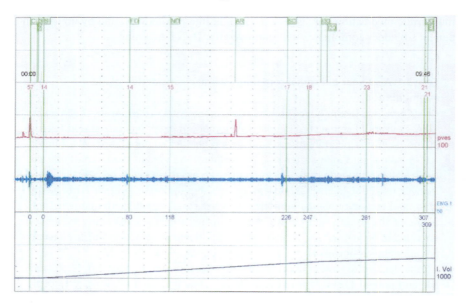

Fig. 3.13 Urodynamic tracing of same patient in Fig. 3.12, 2 months after 200 U onabotulinumtoxinA. The significant improvement in her symptoms coincides with the complete lack of detrusor activity during bladder filling

3.5.6 Adverse Events

The most common adverse events of intravesical BoNT injection are incomplete bladder emptying and urinary tract infections. Urinary tract infections have been reported in 2% to 32% of patients treated, and are usually associated with a large post

3.5 What Are the Results

void residual urine volume (Karsenty et al. 2008). Interestingly, in one series of 30 patients, investigators found that BoNT treatment reduced the incidence of symptomatic urinary tract infections in neurogenic bladder patients by 88% (Game et al. 2008). Although acute urinary retention could also be a problem immediately after injection, the presence of acute retention is usually unrelated to the treatment outcome. The dose of BoNT does, however, appear to be related to the occurrence of a urinary retention (0–33%) or de novo intermittent catheterization (6–88%) (Karsenty et al. 2008). Systemic side effects such as generalized weakness have been reported after bladder injection; however, the incidence is rare and appears to be related to the dose of toxin, or, perhaps, the formulation used (Smith and Chancellor 2004). For example, Grosse and colleagues documented four patients suffering from transient muscle weakness, all after being injected with abobotulinumtoxinA, with symptoms lasting between 2 weeks and 2 months (Grosse et al. 2005). In addition, Del Popolo and associates noted hypothenia in five patients following injection with 1,000 U of abobotulinumtoxinA but the effects were transient, disappearing after 2–4 week (Del Popolo et al. 2008). We have not observed any systemic side effects in the hundreds of patients we have treated with onabotulinumtoxinA over a 10-year period. Other adverse events such as hematuria and injection site pain are generally transient in nature.

Case 3.2: A 41-year-old C6-7 incomplete SCI man with autonomic dysreflexia
Chief Complaint: Frequent headaches, sweating, and the need to catheterize too often.

A 41-year-old man who suffered a C6-7 incomplete SCI after a diving accident 12 years ago is able to self-catheterize but reports sweating and palpitation at a bladder capacity of 150 ml. He is taking antimuscarinic and alpha blocker medication but still has to catheterize himself often and this is interfering significantly with his quality of life.

Urodynamics demonstrated neurogenic detrusor overactivity with detrusor sphincter dyssynergia (Fig. 3.14). The patient's blood pressure increased during the study but with adequate warning the patients vital signs returned to normal after bladder emptying.

The patient requested bladder onabotulinumtoxinA injection and gave his informed consent. The procedure was done in the outpatient clinic. A nurse was present in the procedure room to frequently monitor his vital signs. Two percent lidocaine jelly was infused into the urethra for approximately 5 min and then 40 ml of lidocaine was instilled into the bladder using a 14 French catheter for 10 min (i.e., to prevent autonomic dysreflexia). The procedure was performed at bladder volume of approximately 100–150 ml and the patient remained stable throughout.

Outcome: After about 4 days, the patient noticed significantly less headache and sweating in addition to an increased functional bladder capacity. He was now able to catheterize half as often as before and without experiencing autonomic dysreflexic symptoms (Fig. 3.15). In addition, the patient was able to cut his anticholinergic dose in half. He requested a repeat onabotulinumtoxinA injection in approximately 6 months.

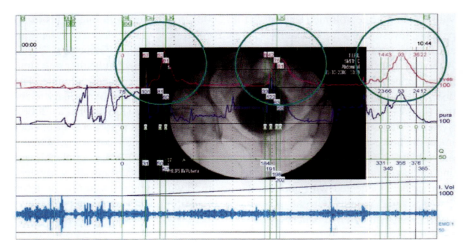

Fig. 3.14 Urodynamic tracing in a 41-year-old man with SCI demonstrating neurogenic detrusor overactivity with detrusor sphincter dyssynergia. The patient has significant incontinence despite being on maximum dose anticholinergic therapy and he complains of autonomic dysreflexia (i.e., elevated blood pressure) during bladder filling

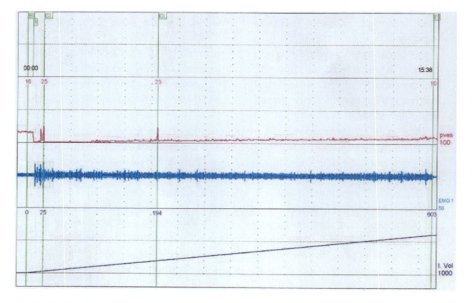

Fig. 3.15 Urodynamic tracing in the same 41-year-old SCI man as in Fig. 3.14, 2 months after bladder injection with 200 U onabotulinumtoxinA. The tracing demonstrates a significant increase in bladder capacity without any detrusor activity. The patient was now able to catheterize less often, reduce his antimuscarinic medication dose by 50%, and was no longer bothered by recurrent episodes of headaches and sweating

3.5.7 Simultaneous Bladder and Sphincter BoNT Injection

We have a small series of patients, both men and women, who were treated with simultaneous bladder and sphincter BoNT injections. The majority had multiple sclerosis while the remaining had thoracic level spinal cord injury. Baseline videourodynamic study documented NDO and DSD and they requested both conditions be treated at one session. Patients were injected with onabotulinumtoxinA, 100–200 U in the sphincter (transurethral in men (200 U) and periurethral in women (100 U)) and 100–200 U in the bladder. Overall, we observed increases in bladder capacity and decreases in residual urine volume. While none of the patients developed de novo stress incontinence, some women's leakage with stress worsened. There was no systemic toxicity seen in this small series with injections into two sites in the genitourinary system. However, only less than a third were able to void adequately and stop self catheterization.

> **Box 3.3: Assessments of American Academy Neurology Therapeutics and Technology Committee**
>
> The American Academy of Neurology Therapeutics and Technology Committee examined clinical studies of BoNT treatment of Neurogenic Detrusor Overactivity (Mauskop and Mathew 2009). A total of two Class I studies, one Class II study, and several Class III studies were evaluated. One Class I study described the safety and efficacy of a single treatment with onabotulinumtoxinA in 59 patients with multiple sclerosis or spinal cord injury (Schurch et al. 2005). The investigators found that BoNT was more effective than placebo in decreasing the frequency of incontinence episodes, improving bladder function, and improving patient quality of life. In a separate Class I study, rimabotulinumtoxinB was used to treat 20 patients with refractory neurogenic or non-neurogenic detrusor overactivity (Ghei et al. 2005). Subjects were followed for 6 weeks and then crossed over to the other treatment paradigm. The study found significant improvements in voided volume, urinary frequency, incontinence episodes, and quality of life parameters in the rimabotulinumtoxinB group compared to placebo. However, the study was limited in several respects. The population study had mixed etiologies of detrusor overactivity (i.e., neurogenic vs. non-neurogenic), follow-up was short and the absence of a washout period and the relatively low dose of rimabotulinumtoxinB used may have biased the results.
>
> In a single Class II study, onabotulinumtoxinA injection was compared to resiniferatoxin instillation (inhibits bladder C-fiber afferent nerves) into the bladder in 25 patients with spinal cord lesions with neurogenic detrusor overactivity (Giannantoni et al. 2004). There was a significant decrease in catheterization and incontinence episodes for both treatments at 6, 12, and 18 months of follow-up. However, the onabotulinumtoxinA injections provided superior clinical and urodynamic benefits as compared to intravesical resiniferatoxin. There were no significant side effects with either treatment. The committee concluded that BoNT is established as safe and effective for the treatment of neurogenic detrusor overactivity in adults (two Class I studies, one Class II study). It further recommended that BoNT should be offered as a treatment option for neurogenic detrusor overactivity (Level A).

Case 3.3: A 54-year-old multiple sclerosis woman with urgency incontinence
Chief Complaint: Urgency and urgency incontinence but cannot tolerate antimuscarinics.

A 54-year-old ambulatory woman with an 8-year history of chronic progressive multiple sclerosis (MS) presents with urgency, nocturia × 3, and approximately two episodes of urgency incontinence daily requiring the use of large absorbent diapers. She tried several oral antimuscarinics but had severe dry mouth and constipation. More importantly, she developed urinary retention with a trial of oxybutynin in the past and was unable to perform self-catheterization due to lack of manual dexterity in her hands and spasticity in her legs. In addition, her neurologist wanted to avoid drugs with anticholinergic side effects given her mild cognitive changes.

Urodynamics revealed neurogenic detrusor overactivity without detrusor sphincter dyssynergia. Her post-void residual was 30 ml.

Treatment: The patient was highly motivated to request onabotulinumtoxinA bladder injection as she had friends who had significant improvement in their muscle spasticity with BoNT injection. After informed consent where she understood and accepted the risk of retention and need for catheterization, 100 U of onabotulinumtoxinA was injected in ten sites, mostly trigone and via the submucosal technique in order to minimize the dose and localize the response.

Outcome: Fortunately, the patient did not develop retention although her residual volume increased to 70 ml. She did report a marked decrease in day and night time frequency, sensation of urgency and frequency of urgency incontinence. While she still experiences nocturia × 1, and occasional urge incontinence episodes (1–2 times/week), her quality of life has dramatically improved with onabotulinumtoxinA bladder injection. The improvement lasted for 9 months before she requested a repeat injection. She wanted to have the 100 U dose again because, although not completely dry, she did not want to risk urinary retention with using higher dosages of onabotulinumtoxinA.

3.6 Future Perspective: Electrical Neuromodulation and Stem Cell Research

Functional electrical stimulation is a valuable tool used in various medical fields to induce muscle activation, walking, and even bladder control. For the bladder, modulation and stimulation of sacral nerve roots can provide an alternative treatment option in patients with voiding dysfunction and chronic pelvic pain. Results of using sacral nerve modulators in refractory urgency and urgency incontinence been reported for NDO (Chartier-Kastler et al. 2000). Exciting research is currently underway that may selectively turn off the sphincter and turn on the bladder based on the site and the frequency of nerve stimulation. There is much research using stem cells to regenerate the spinal cord and/or peripheral nerves in spinal cord injury patients. This hope is one reason why some spinal cord injury patients are glad to have twice a year BoNT injection rather than surgical augmentation because they believe they will be able to urinate again with their own bladder if stem cell research cures spinal cord injury.

3.7 Conclusions

It has been over a decade since we started using botulinum toxin in selected patients with refractory neurogenic detrusor overactivity and in registered clinical trials of onabotulinumtoxinA for neurogenic detrusor. We have seen remarkable improvement in bladder function when high doses of anticholinergics simply are not enough. Many of our patients have done well over the years with a simple outpatient injection of botulinum toxin and have been spared from more invasive reconstructive surgery. Although we are aware of and look out for systemic toxicity and antibody formation, neither of us has seen it in any of our neurogenic detrusor overactivity patients.

References

Chancellor MB (2010) Ten years single surgeon experience with botulinum toxin in the urinary tract; clinical observations and research discovery. Int Urol Nephrol 42(2):383–391

Chancellor MB, Patel V, Leng W, Shenot P, Lam W, Chapple C (2011) OnabotulinumtoxinA in patients with urinary incontinence due to neurogenic detrusor overactivity: effects on health related quality of life. 2011 American Urological Association Annual Meeting. May 2011, Abstract1518.

Chartier-Kastler EJ, Mongiat-Artus P, Bitker MO, Chancellor MB, Richard F, Denys P (2000) Long-term results of augmentation cystoplasty in spinal cord injury patients. Spinal Cord 38(8):490–494

Coelho A, Dinis P, Pinto R, Gorgal T, Silva C, Silva A, Silva J, Cruz CD, Cruz F, Avelino A (2009) Distribution of the high-affinity binding site and intracellular target of botulinum toxin type A in the human bladder. Eur Urol 57(5):884–890

Comperat E, Reitz A, Delcourt A, Capron F, Denys P, Chartier-Kastler E (2006) Histologic features in the urinary bladder wall affected from neurogenic overactivity – a comparison of inflammation, oedema and fibrosis with and without injection of botulinum toxin type A. Eur Urol 50(5):1058–1064

de Paiva A, Meunier FA, Molgo J, Aoki KR, Dolly JO (1999) Functional repair of motor endplates after botulinum neurotoxin type A poisoning: biphasic switch of synaptic activity between nerve sprouts and their parent terminals. Proc Natl Acad Sci USA 96(6):3200–3205

Del Popolo G, Filocamo MT, Li Marzi V, Macchiarella A, Cecconi F, Lombardi G, Nicita G (2008) Neurogenic detrusor overactivity treated with English botulinum toxin A: 8-year experience of one single centre. Eur Urol 53(5):1013–1019

Ehren I, Volz D, Farrelly E, Berglund L, Brundin L, Hultling C, Lafolie P (2007) Efficacy and impact of botulinum toxin A on quality of life in patients with neurogenic detrusor overactivity: a randomised, placebo-controlled, double-blind study. Scand J Urol Nephrol 41(4):335–340

Eleopra R, Tugnoli V, Rossetto O, De Grandis D, Montecucco C (1998) Different time courses of recovery after poisoning with botulinum neurotoxin serotypes A and E in humans. Neurosci Lett 256(3):135–138

Foran PG, Mohammed N, Lisk GO, Nagwaney S, Lawrence GW, Johnson E, Smith L, Aoki KR, Dolly JO (2003) Evaluation of the therapeutic usefulness of botulinum neurotoxin B, C1, E, and F compared with the long lasting type A. Basis for distinct durations of inhibition of exocytosis in central neurons. J Biol Chem 278(2):1363–1371

Fowler CJ (2007) Update on the neurology of Parkinson's disease. Neurourol Urodyn 26(1):103–109

Game X, Castel-Lacanal E, Bentaleb Y, Thiry-Escudie I, De Boissezon X, Malavaud B, Marque P, Rischmann P (2008) Botulinum toxin A detrusor injections in patients with neurogenic detrusor overactivity significantly decrease the incidence of symptomatic urinary tract infections. Eur Urol 53(3):613–618

Ghei M, Maraj BH, Miller R, Nathan S, O'Sullivan C, Fowler CJ, Shah PJ, Malone-Lee J (2005) Effects of botulinum toxin B on refractory detrusor overactivity: a randomized, double-blind, placebo controlled, crossover trial. J Urol 174(5):1873–1877; discussion 1877

Giannantoni A, Di Stasi SM, Stephen RL, Bini V, Costantini E, Porena M (2004) Intravesical resiniferatoxin versus botulinum-A toxin injections for neurogenic detrusor overactivity: a prospective randomized study. J Urol 172(1):240–243

Giannantoni A, Rossi A, Mearini E, Del Zingaro M, Porena M, Berardelli A (2009) Botulinum toxin A for overactive bladder and detrusor muscle overactivity in patients with Parkinson's disease and multiple system atrophy. J Urol 182(4):1453–1457

Ginsberg D, Gousse A, Keppenne V, Sievert KD, Thompson C, Lam W, Jenkins B, Haag Molkenteller C (2011) Phase 3 efficacy and safety study of onabotulinumtoxinA in patients with urinary incontinence due to neurogenic detrusor overactivity. 2011 American Urological Association Annual Meeting. May 2011, Abstract 1515.

Grosse J, Kramer G, Stohrer M (2005) Success of repeat detrusor injections of botulinum a toxin in patients with severe neurogenic detrusor overactivity and incontinence. Eur Urol 47(5):653–659

Haferkamp A, Schurch B, Reitz A, Krengel U, Grosse J, Kramer G, Schumacher S, Bastian PJ, Buttner R, Muller SC, Stohrer M (2004) Lack of ultrastructural detrusor changes following endoscopic injection of botulinum toxin type a in overactive neurogenic bladder. Eur Urol 46(6):784–791

Jankovic J, Vuong KD, Ahsan J (2003) Comparison of efficacy and immunogenicity of original versus current botulinum toxin in cervical dystonia. Neurology 60(7):1186–1188

Kalsi V, Apostolidis A, Gonzales G, Elneil S, Dasgupta P, Fowler CJ (2008) Early effect on the overactive bladder symptoms following botulinum neurotoxin type A injections for detrusor overactivity. Eur Urol 54(1):181–187

Kaplan SA, Chancellor MB, Blaivas JG (1991) Bladder and sphincter behavior in patients with spinal cord lesions. J Urol 146(1):113–117

Karsenty G, Denys P, Amarenco G, De Seze M, Game X, Haab F, Kerdraon J, Perrouin-Verbe B, Ruffion A, Saussine C, Soler JM, Schurch B, Chartier-Kastler E (2008) Botulinum toxin A (botox) intradetrusor injections in adults with neurogenic detrusor overactivity/neurogenic overactive bladder: a systematic literature review. Eur Urol 53(2):275–287

Karsenty G, Elzayat E, Delapparent T, St-Denis B, Lemieux MC, Corcos J (2007) Botulinum toxin type a injections into the trigone to treat idiopathic overactive bladder do not induce vesicoureteral reflux. J Urol 177(3):1011–1014

Keller JE, Neale EA (2001) The role of the synaptic protein snap-25 in the potency of botulinum neurotoxin type A. J Biol Chem 276(16):13476–13482

Keller JE, Neale EA, Oyler G, Adler M (1999) Persistence of botulinum neurotoxin action in cultured spinal cord cells. FEBS Lett 456(1):137–142

Klaphajone J, Kitisomprayoonkul W, Sriplakit S (2005) Botulinum toxin type A injections for treating neurogenic detrusor overactivity combined with low-compliance bladder in patients with spinal cord lesions. Arch Phys Med Rehabil 86(11):2114–2118

Kuo HC (2007) Comparison of effectiveness of detrusor, suburothelial and bladder base injections of botulinum toxin a for idiopathic detrusor overactivity. J Urol 178(4 Pt 1):1359–1363

Mauskop A, Mathew N (2009) Assessment: botulinum neurotoxin in the treatment of autonomic disorders and pain (an evidence-based review): report of the therapeutics and technology assessment subcommittee of the American academy of neurology. Neurology 72(15):1367; author reply 1367–1368

Mehnert U, Boy S, Schmid M, Reitz A, von Hessling A, Hodler J, Schurch B (2009) A morphological evaluation of botulinum neurotoxin A injections into the detrusor muscle using magnetic resonance imaging. World J Urol 27(3):397–403

Pinto R, Lopes T, Frias B, Silva A, Silva JA, Silva CM, Cruz C, Cruz F, Dinis P (2010) Trigonal injection of botulinum toxin A in patients with refractory bladder pain syndrome/interstitial cystitis. Eur Urol 58(3):360–365

Schmid DM, Sauermann P, Werner M, Schuessler B, Blick N, Muentener M, Strebel RT, Perucchini D, Scheiner D, Schaer G, John H, Reitz A, Hauri D, Schurch B (2006) Experience with 100 cases treated with botulinum-A toxin injections in the detrusor muscle for idiopathic overactive bladder syndrome refractory to anticholinergics. J Urol 176(1):177–185

Schulte-Baukloh H, Bigalke H, Miller K, Heine G, Pape D, Lehmann J, Knispel HH (2008) Botulinum neurotoxin type A in urology: antibodies as a cause of therapy failure. Int J Urol 15(5):407–415; discussion 415

Schulte-Baukloh H, Michael T, Schobert J, Stolze T, Knispel HH (2002) Efficacy of botulinum-a toxin in children with detrusor hyperreflexia due to myelomeningocele: preliminary results. Urology 59(3):325–327; discussion 327–328

Schurch B, de Seze M, Denys P, Chartier-Kastler E, Haab F, Everaert K, Plante P, Perrouin-Verbe B, Kumar C, Fraczek S, Brin MF (2005) Botulinum toxin type a is a safe and effective treatment for neurogenic urinary incontinence: results of a single treatment, randomized, placebo controlled 6-month study. J Urol 174(1):196–200

Schurch B, Stohrer M, Kramer G, Schmid DM, Gaul G, Hauri D (2000) Botulinum-A toxin for treating detrusor hyperreflexia in spinal cord injured patients: a new alternative to anticholinergic drugs? Preliminary results. J Urol 164(3 Pt 1):692–697

Sloop RR, Cole BA, Escutin RO (1997) Human response to botulinum toxin injection: type B compared with type A. Neurology 49(1):189–194

Smith CP, Chancellor MB (2004) Emerging role of botulinum toxin in the management of voiding dysfunction. J Urol 171(6 Pt 1):2128–2137

Smith CP, Chancellor MB (2005) Simplified bladder botulinum-toxin delivery technique using flexible cystoscope and 10 sites of injection. J Endourol 19(7):880–882

Smith CP, Nishiguchi J, O'Leary M, Yoshimura N, Chancellor MB (2005) Single-institution experience in 110 patients with botulinum toxin A injection into bladder or urethra. Urology 65(1):37–41

Winge K, Skau AM, Stimpel H, Nielsen KK, Werdelin L (2006) Prevalence of bladder dysfunction in Parkinsons disease. Neurourol Urodyn 25(2):116–122

Woodside JR, McGuire EJ (1979) Urethral hypotonicity after suprasacral spinal cord injury. J Urol 121(6):783–785

Yalla SV, Blunt KJ, Fam BA, Constantinople NL, Gittes RF (1977) Detrusor-urethral sphincter dyssynergia. J Urol 118(6):1026–1029

Overactive Bladder and Idiopathic Detrusor Overactivity

4.1 Introduction

Overactive bladder (OAB), estimated to afflict up to 33 million Americans, (Stewart et al. 2003) is a condition resulting in a disruption to the normal micturition process. It is a syndrome complex characterized by urinary urgency, frequency and may or may not be accompanied by incontinence. Incontinence is due to involuntary contraction of the detrusor muscle during bladder filling (detrusor overactivity). Most cases of incontinence arise without obvious pathology. In such cases, abnormal bladder muscle contractions are termed idiopathic detrusor overactivity (IDO). A smaller number of cases are secondary to neurogenic pathology and are termed neurogenic detrusor overactivity (Chap. 3).

4.2 Rationale for BoNT Use in Idiopathic OAB

Common pharmacologic treatments to reduce bladder contractility include anticholinergics, antispasmodics, and tricyclic antidepressants. However, these therapies are associated with a high incidence of side effects including dry mouth, constipation and blurred vision, and often are not effective enough to reduce incontinence in cases of severe overactivity. Newer agents that target sensory fibers (e.g., capsaicin and resiniferatoxin) have shown early clinical promise although larger studies are still needed to judge the overall efficacy of this approach (Chancellor and de Groat 1999). Currently, the only options available to patients who do not respond to or discontinue anticholinergic therapy are invasive procedures such as implantable devices to chronically stimulate the sacral nerve or surgical bladder augmentation. While these procedures may be effective for some patients, they are highly invasive, do not necessarily guarantee continence, and may have long term complications (Bosch 1998; Hohenfellner et al. 2000; Van Kerrebroeck et al. 1997).

Recently, studies have been carried out using botulinum neurotoxin (BoNT) in the treatment of patients who suffer from bladder overactivity. Suppression of involuntary detrusor contractions has been attempted via the local administration of

BoNT serotype A to the detrusor muscle, which inhibits acetylcholine release by cleaving SNAP 25, a protein integral to successful docking and release of vesicles within the nerve endings, including acetylcholine, calcitonin gene-related peptides (CGRP), glutamate and substance-P (Blasi et al. 1993; Cui et al. 2004; Meunier et al. 1996; Welch et al. 2000). BoNT is believed to inhibit the acetylcholine-mediated detrusor contractions and may also inhibit other vesical-bound neurotransmitters in both the afferent and efferent pathways of the bladder wall, urothelium, or lamina propria (Chancellor et al. 2008).

4.3 How to Do It

It should be emphasized that no standardized injection technique exists for BoNT injection in lower urinary tract tissues. For patients with idiopathic detrusor overactivity and OAB, onabotulinumtoxinA doses have ranged from 100 to 300 units. However, few controlled studies have been performed to determine the optimum dose or toxin dilution in idiopathic detrusor overactivity patient populations. Different injection paradigms have been described (i.e., trigone vs. trigone-sparing) although none has been proven to be superior to the other. In addition, fear of inducing vesicoureteral reflux with trigonal injection was disproven in a study by Karsenty and colleagues (Karsenty et al. 2007). Bladder injections with BoNT can be made using either a rigid or flexible cystoscope, under general or local anesthesia.

4.3.1 Simplified Delivery Using Flexible Cystoscope

Patients are treated in an outpatient setting after local anesthetization with intraurethral 2% lidocaine jelly and 30 ml of intravesical 1–2% lidocaine for 10–15 min. Using a 25–27 gauge, disposable flexible injection needle (Olympus Inc., Melville, NY) inserted through a flexible cystoscope, 100 units of onabotulinumtoxinA (Allergan Inc., Irvine, CA) diluted in 10 ml of preservative-free saline, is injected submucosally into ten sites within the bladder trigone and base (Fig. 4.1). This injection technique is a modification of our 30–40-site injection technique previously described in treating patients with neurogenic or overactive bladders and can be completely performed within a 15-min office procedure time slot (Smith and Chancellor 2004). All patients receive peri-operative oral antibiotics and are followed up subjectively by either phone or office interview in addition to post-void residual measurement with bladder ultrasound during clinic visits.

Ten patients with refractory idiopathic OAB have been treated utilizing this novel technique. Subjective improvement rates are similar to our prior reported rates of approximately 80% in NDO patients using 30 sites of injection (Smith and Chancellor 2005). Patients begin seeing effects of the treatment 7–10 days after injection with durable responses lasting between 3 and 6 months. In comparison to use of a more widespread injection technique (e.g., 30–40 injections

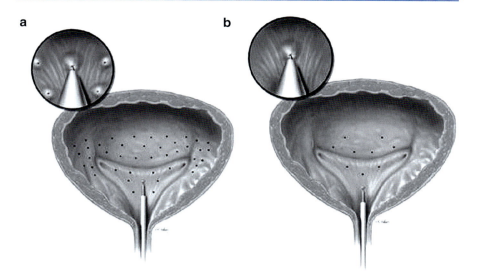

Fig. 4.1 Diagram depicting botulinum toxin injection sites within the detrusor muscle of the bladder. In contrast to other investigators, we target the trigone because of its rich sensory innervation. However, we avoid injecting the dome of the bladder to prevent inadvertent bowel perforation. The panel on the *left* depicts our 30–40 injection template utilized for neurogenic or severe idiopathic overactive bladder patients and typically 200–300 units of onabotulinumtoxinA injection. In contrast, the *right panel* describes the paradigm we use in mild to moderate idiopathic overactive bladder patients or patients with interstitial cystitis using 100 units of onabotulinumtoxinA (Copyright obtained Smith and Chancellor 2005)

throughout bladder excluding the dome) or using higher toxin dosages (e.g., 200 U onabotulinumtoxinA), no patient has developed urinary retention or elevated post-void residual following our modified injection technique.

Prior studies have shown that maximal toxin effect is dependent on toxin dose and distribution (Kim et al. 2003). In our personal experience, we have noted several patients with OAB develop elevated post-void residuals or even frank urinary retention using our originally described injection technique (Smith and Chancellor 2004). By reducing toxin dosage and distribution but still targeting dense sensory and motor innervation in the trigone and bladder neck, we have successfully treated refractory OAB patients with our modified injection technique. Moreover, the 10-point injection technique is fast and efficient and amenable as an outpatient procedure utilizing a flexible cystoscope. The 27-gauge flexible injection needle has excellent piercing capability and a stopper on the tip of the sheath to maintain proper needle length that allow or reliable and controlled toxin injection into bladder submucosal tissues (Fig. 4.2). Moreover, the needle is pre-sterilized and disposable, which will help allay fears of cross-contamination.

Fig. 4.2 Photograph of the flexible cystoscope with injection needle extended from the needle sheath

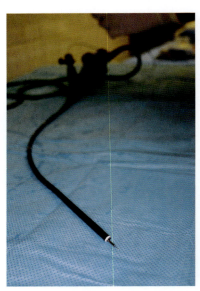

4.3.2 Depth of Injection

Many questions arise regarding how deep to inject the toxin: intramuscular, submucosal, or epithelial. Mehnert and colleagues performed a study where neurogenic detrusor overactive (NDO) patient's bladders were injected intramuscularly with 300 units of onabotulinumtoxinA mixed with gadolinium (Mehnert et al. 2009). Immediately following injection, patients underwent an MRI study to document the distribution of the gadolinium. The investigators found that almost 18% of injected onabotulinumtoxinA was localized outside the bladder wall in the extraperitoneal fat. In addition, Kuo demonstrated significant increases in functional bladder capacity, significant reductions in urge episodes, without an increase in post-void residual in patients with idiopathic overactive bladder undergoing bladder trigone suburothelial injections compared to patients injected intramuscularly outside of the trigonal area (Kuo 2007). Unfortunately, without the ability to label BoNT to identify exactly where it localizes within the bladder, it is impossible to define differences in toxin distribution with various injection paradigms.

Our goal with bladder injections is to minimize the number of injections required by maximizing spread while preventing migration of the toxin into the retroperitoneal space (Fig. 4.3). Figure 4.3 Panel B shows what we would consider "poor" injection technique. The needle placement is too shallow creating a blistering effect of the urothelium with loss of vascular markings and minimal toxin spread. As the needle is inserted further (Fig. 4.3, Panel C) the injection is then directed submucosally with significant elevation of the mucosal wall in both vertical and horizontal planes and persistence of mucosal vascular markings. We consider Panel C as a "good" injection technique. In addition, because we have avoided intramuscular injection, our risk of extravesical extravasation is mitigated.

Fig. 4.3 Photograph illustrating differences in the depth of BoNT injection. *Panel A* shows pre-injection bladder following needle entry. *Panel B* demonstrates superficial needle placement with epithelial injection. Notice the blanching of the urothelium with loss of vascular markings. *Panel C* displays the desired depth of submucosal injection as the needle is inserted further. A greater spread of toxin is noted without loss of vascular markings

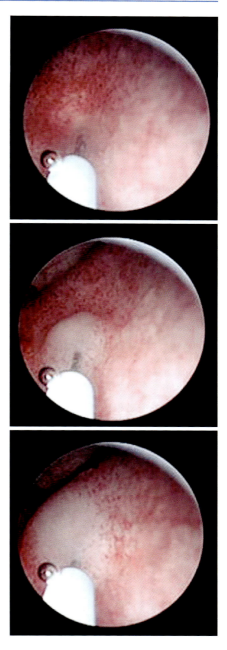

Case Study 4.1: A 55-year-old woman with retention after BoNT injection

Chief Complaint: Refractory urgency, frequency, and urgency incontinence.

Presentation: A 55 year-old woman is highly bothered for over 20 years with worsening daily urinary urgency, urinary frequency of over 14 episodes per day and almost daily small episode of urgency incontinence. She has tried antimuscarinics without relief. She was previously diagnosed with interstitial cystitis and tried various bladder cocktail instillations without any benefit. She tried percutaneous neuromodulation without improvement.

Pertinent Exam and Evaluation: Physical exam revealed no suprapubic tenderness or abdominal masses. Pelvic exam was normal. Cystometrogram documented an involuntary detrusor contraction at 90 ml that she was able to inhibit and not leak but she developed a second involuntary contraction at 134 ml which she could not inhibit and had a large leak episode (Fig. 4.4a). Her bladder was slowly refilled to 200 ml and asked to cough but did not develop stress urinary incontinence. Voiding cystogram demonstrated bilateral grade II vesicoureteral reflux (Fig. 4.5). Her post void residual urine was less than 25 ml.

Treatment: Patient had previous cosmetic BoNT and was interested in bladder botulinum toxin. After explaining that bladder injection of botulinum toxin for overactive bladder is off-label and after describing the various potential risks, the patient had time to ask questions, gave informed consent and requested scheduling. The procedure was done in the office with local anesthesia. The procedure was done about 5 years ago where we typically used 200 U onabotulinumtoxinA as our initial dose. She was injected throughout the bladder in 1 ml aliquots with 200 U onabotulinumtoxinA diluted in 20 ml of sterile saline.

Outcome: Within 7 days, the patient noted less urgency and frequency but also need to strain to void. Her residual urine was measured at 215 ml. She was taught clean intermittent self-catheterization that she decided to do twice a day, once in morning and once at night since she can still void on her own. Her urgency incontinence resolved but she had to self-catheterize for about 12 weeks at which time she reported her residual urine was consistent below 100 ml. Figure 4.4b, c cystometrograms after her 1st and 2nd BoNT injections, respectively. The patient was not able to void despite straining to a capacity of nearly 500 ml after the 1st 200 U onabotulinumtoxinA injection (Fig. 4.4b). She was able to generate voluntary voiding contraction after 2nd 100 U onabotulinumtoxinA injection (Fig. 4.4c).

She continued to notice clinical improvement for 8 months at which time she started to notice episodes of incontinence. Her residual urine volume at that time was 25 ml. She was worried about having retention again and having to catheterize herself. But she was very pleased with the profound change in her micturition pattern and gaining bladder control after so many years. She asked for repeat injection and we mutually decided on using 100 U onabotulinumtoxinA. Her second injection was ten submucosal sites at the bladder base and trigone of 1 ml aliquots with 100 U onabotulinumtoxinA dissolved in 10 ml of sterile saline. She noticed similar improvement in her voiding symptoms and resolution of incontinence but did not notice the sensation of incomplete emptying or straining to void. Her residual urine remained in 50–70 ml range without infection or need to restart the self-catheterization. The efficacy of the 2nd injection also lasted about 8 months.

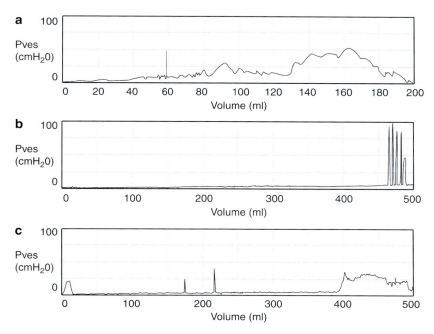

Fig. 4.4 Cystometrograms before BoNT injection (**a**), after 1st 200 U onabotulinumtoxinA injection (**b**), and after 2nd 100 U onabotulinumtoxinA injection (**c**). Prior to BoNT cystometrogram demonstrated an involuntary detrusor contraction at 90 and 134 ml (**a**). The patient was not able to void despite straining at a capacity of nearly 500 ml after the 1st 200 U onabotulinumtoxinA injection (**b**). She was able to generate voluntary voiding contraction at approximately 400 ml after 2nd 100 U onabotulinumtoxinA injection (**c**)

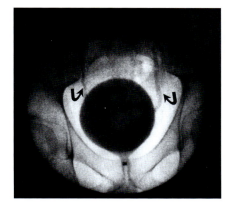

Fig. 4.5 Voiding cystogram demonstrated bilateral grade II vesicoureteral reflux (*arrows*)

4.4 What Are the Results?

4.4.1 Botulium Toxin Type A

Sahai and colleagues detailed the first randomized placebo-controlled trial comparing the effect of 200 U of onabotulinumtoxinA versus saline bladder injection in 34 patients (i.e., 16 onabotulinumtoxinA and 18 placebo) with idiopathic detrusor overactivity and inadequately treated with 6 months of anticholinergic therapy (Sahai et al. 2007). A total of 200 U of onabotulinumtoxinA was diluted in 20 ml of saline (i.e., 10 U/ml; or saline was used alone as placebo) and was injected in 20 places within the bladder wall, sparing the trigone. The primary endpoint measure was change in maximum cystometric capacity. OnabotulinumtoxinA improved maximum cystometric capacity significantly by 96 ml at 12 weeks. In addition, marked reductions in urinary frequency, and decreases in the number of urge urinary incontinence episodes and in the level of urgency was observed. The investigators also noted improvements in quality of life questionnaires in the onabotulinumtoxinA treated group.

Brubaker and associates compared the effects of 200 U of onabotulinumtoxinA versus saline bladder injections in 43 female patients with refractory urge urinary incontinence defined as >6 incontinence episodes/3 days and having failed at least two anticholinergic drugs (Brubaker et al. 2008). Patients were randomized in a 2:1 ratio: 28 patients received 200 U of onabotulinumtoxinA diluted in 6 ml of preservative free saline (i.e., 33 U/ml) and 15 patients received saline injections alone. A total of 15–20 injections were placed in the posterior wall of the bladder sparing the trigone. The primary endpoint was time to failure, defined as a patient global impression of improvement score of 4 or greater 2 months after treatment. Sixty percent of patients treated with onabotulinumtoxinA demonstrated improvements in patient global impression of improvement score with a median duration of response of 373 days compared to 62 days or less for the placebo group. In addition, patients treated with onabotulinumtoxinA displayed greater than a 75% reduction in urge incontinence episodes by 3 day voiding diary (Fig. 4.6). Unfortunately, the study was curtailed after recruiting 43 patients because 43% of patients treated with onabotulinumtoxinA required intermittent catheterization for a median duration of approximately 2 months.

Flynn and colleague evaluated the effect of two doses of onabotulinumtoxinA (i.e., 200 U and 300 U) versus placebo in 22 patients with refractory OAB defined as: greater than 2 daily urge incontinence episodes/day on a 3 day voiding diary, a 24 h pad weight of >100 g, and failure to respond to at least one anticholinergic medication (Flynn et al. 2009). Candidates did not require urodynamically proven overactivity to be included in this study. The investigators were blinded to the dose of toxin given at the time of the study, thus the onabotulinumtoxinA results represent the combined results of both doses (i.e., 15 patients treated with onabotulinumtoxinA and 7 patients treated with placebo). The primary endpoints analyzed were the number of incontinence episodes/24 h and the quality of life and urinary distress

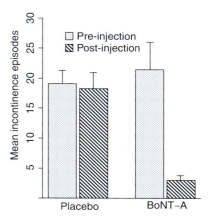

Fig. 4.6 Note the dramatic decrease in urge incontinent episodes by 3 day voiding diary in idiopathic detrusor overactivity patients treated with 200 U of onabotulinumtoxinA. Interestingly, as opposed to anticholinergic trials, no placebo effect was observed (Copyright obtained from Brubaker et al. 2008)

questionnaire results. Interestingly, as opposed to the two prior studies, these investigators diluted onabotulinumtoxinA in only 3 ml (i.e., 66–100 U/ml) and injected the bladder in 10–12 sites along the posterior bladder wall, sparing the trigone. At 6 weeks of follow-up, significant reductions in incontinence episodes/day were noted in the onabotulinumtoxinA treated group (i.e., 57.5%). In addition, marked improvements in quality of life and urinary distress symptoms scores were observed as well. Furthermore, pad weight decreased by 45% and the mean number of pads/day dropped from 4.4 to 2.2 pads/day.

The largest and most recent randomized placebo-controlled study evaluated several doses of onabotulinumtoxinA (i.e., 50, 100, 150, 200, and 300 U) versus placebo in 313 patients with idiopathic OAB and urinary urge incontinence not adequately managed with anticholinergic medications (Dmochowski et al. 2010). Patients had to experience at least eight urinary urge incontinence episodes/week and eight or more micturitions/day to be included in the study. The primary endpoint was weekly urinary urgency incontinence episodes at 12 weeks. Subjects were injected at 20 sites into the detrusor muscle (i.e., 0.5 ml/site) avoiding the trigone and the dome. The authors stated that significant difference from placebo was observed in the number of urgency incontinence episodes/week at many time points. However, they also stated that a clear dose response effect was not observed in regards to efficacy, although by non-parametric analysis minimal additional benefit was achieved by doses above 150 U of onabotulinumtoxinA. In contrast, a clear dose response relationship was displayed in the proportion of patients with a post-treatment residual urine volume of 200 ml or greater.

4.4.1.1 Meta-Analysis

Anger and colleagues performed a meta-analysis of the three randomized, placebo-controlled trials up to that time point using onabotulinumtoxinA in patients with idiopathic OAB (Anger et al. 2010). Pooled analysis of the three studies revealed that patients treated with onabotulinumtoxinA had almost four fewer episodes of urge urinary incontinence per day than placebo treated patients (Fig. 4.7). Their

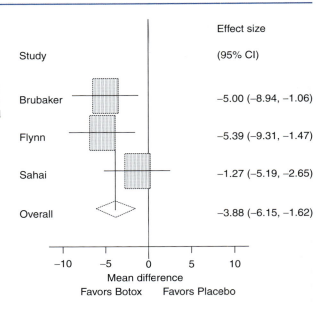

Fig. 4.7 Pooled analysis from three randomized clinical trials estimating the reduction in urge incontinence episodes per day in onabotulinumtoxinA treated compared to placebo treated patients (Copyright obtained from Anger et al. 2010)

analysis also revealed that onabotulinumtoxinA treated patient's demonstrated improved quality of life scores, estimated by a 15 point drop in urinary distress inventory (UDI-6) scores compared to placebo injected patients. However, the benefit from onabotulinumtoxinA was curbed by the nearly ninefold increase in the risk of elavated post-void residual urine volume in onabotulinumtoxinA treated patients compared to controls.

A recent European expert panel report gave BoNT the highest grade level recommendation (i.e., grade A) for the treatment of refractory idiopathic detrusor overactivity (Apostolidis et al. 2009). Guidance regarding the technique for injection was more ambiguous given the lack of literature addressing this topic (Table 4.1).

4.4.2 Botulinum Toxin Type B

RimabotulinumtoxinB has also been utilized in the OAB population and its effects were described in a study of 15 patients treated with detrusor injections. (Popat et al. 2005) Investigators found that 14 of 15 patients responded to rimabotulinumtoxinB treatment with a mean decrease in daily micturition episodes of 5.27 ($p < 0.001$). Interestingly, the duration of response lasted between 19 and 98 days and was correlated to toxin dose (e.g., 2,500–15,000 U). However, even the longest response to rimabotulinumtoxinB injection was of shorter duration than the 6-month subjective and objective responses to onabotulinumtoxinA injection demonstrated in neurogenic and idiopathic detrusor overactivity. Their results suggest that BoNT serotype A may be a more durable treatment than serotype B for detrusor overactivity.

Table 4.1 European panel of experts level of recommendations for BoNT use in patients with overactivity bladder and idiopathic detrusor overactivity

Idiopathic detrusor overactivity and overactive bladder	Grade
Use BoNT to treat refractory idiopathic detrusor overactivity in patients willing to use clean intermittent catheterization. Use caution because the risk of voiding difficulty as well as the duration of effect has not been accurately evaluated to date. Future studies should address the benefit-risk ratio for the best minimal dosage.	A
All patients should accept in writing the possible need to perform clean intermittent catheterization following treatment.	A
Residual volumes should be measured regularly for the first month starting at the first week.	A
Patients should be told that the treatment does not last indefinitely but has a mean duration of 6 months.	A
Comparison of injection techniques	
The dilution of onabotulinumtoxinA should be 10 U/ml per site: thus, the number of injection sites depends on the total dosage being administered (i.e., 30 sites for a dosage of onabotulinumtoxinA 300 U in neurogenic detrusor overactivity). The optimum dose for dilution of abobotulinumtoxinA has yet to be established.[a]	B
The choice of flexible or rigid cystoscope should be left to local expertise.	C
The depth and location for injections should be within the detrusor muscle outside the trigone.	C

Adapted from Apostolidis et al. 2009
The most typical dose we use to treat idiopathic OAB is 100 U of onabotulinumtoxinA and for neurogenic detrusor overactivity is 200 U of onabotulinumtoxinA

4.4.3 Predictors of Poor Response

Sahai and colleagues performed pre and post urodynamic testing in 34 patients with IDO and treated with 200 U of onabotulinumtoxinA to identify potential predictors of poor response (Sahai et al. 2008). The investigators found significantly higher baseline maximum detrusor pressure in patients non-responsive to onabotulinumtoxinA. They suggested a maximum detrusor pressure of greater than 110 cmH20 as predictive of a poor response to 200 U of onabotulinumtoxinA. In contrast, Cohen and associates could find no preoperative demographic or urodynamic parameters to predict successful treatment with 100–150 U of onabotulinumtoxinA in their cohort of idiopathic OAB patients (Cohen et al. 2009).

> **Case Study 4.2: A 72-year-old man with refractory lower urinary tract symptoms but could not tolerate antimuscarinics**
> *Chief Complaint:* Urgency, frequency, and nocturia
>   A 72-year-old man underwent transurethral microwave therapy for irritative and obstructive voiding symptoms two and half years ago. Patient reported improved

flow rate but had persistent urinary frequency, urgency, and four episodes of nocturia per night despite fluid restriction after dinner. He tried two alpha blockers without improvement. He was prescribed three brands of antimuscarinics and had dry mouth and constipation with the pills. His wife was worried about taking an anticholinergic agent as the patient is being evaluated by a geriatrician for mild cognitive deficiencies. Patient has a history of cardiac pacemaker implantation and noted that his cardiologist told him his heart was doing well.

Pertinent Exam and Evaluation: On physical exam, the patient had a 25 g prostate with no nodules. The remaining genitourinary system was normal. His PSA was 2.2. During uroflow studies the patient voided 165 ml with a maximum flow rate of 15 ml/s and a residual urine volume of 22 ml. Cystometrogram noted no involuntary detrusor contraction but a maximal cystometric capacity of 195 ml and a maximum detrusor voiding pressure of 62 cmH20.

Treatment: The patient reported significant decreased quality of life and wanted to try botulinum toxin bladder injection. Risks were explained to the patient and informed consent was obtained. The patient underwent flexible cystoscopy with onabotulinumtoxinA injection to the bladder trigone and base in ten sites (100 U/10 ml). The procedure was done in the office with local anesthesia.

Outcome: Within a week, the patient noted a decrease in his nocturia. At one month follow-up, the patient reported less frequency and urgency and now gets up about once to twice a night. He did not report any difficulty voiding and think his flow is "strong." Uroflow noted voided volume of 258 ml with a maximum flow rate of 14.2 ml/s and a residual urine volume of 54 ml. The man noted symptomatic improvement for 6 months with his first injection and 10 months after the 2nd injection that he requested.

4.5　Side Effects

A significant number of patients with IDO would probably decline BoNT treatment if there was a high risk of long-term catheterization. Surprisingly, Popat et al. described de novo self-catheterization rates as high as 69% in patients with neurogenic overactive bladder and 19% in patients with idiopathic overactive bladder after injection of 300 U and 200 U of onabotulinumtoxinA, respectively (Popat et al. 2005). In addition, Kessler et al. described de novo catheterization rates of 45% in patients with idiopathic or neurogenic overactive bladder following detrusor injection of 300 U of onabotulinumtoxinA (Kessler et al. 2005).

The high rates of self-catheterization observed in some series might be explained by differences in what each study defines as a clinically relevant postvoid residual >100 mL in the study by Popat et al. versus >150 mL in the study by Kessler et al. (Kessler et al. 2005; Popat et al. 2005). However, two other series reported low post-injection post void residual urine volume of 15 mL and 47 mL after injection of 300 U and 100–300 U of onabotulinumtoxinA, respectively (Schulte-Baukloh et al.

4.5 Side Effects

2005b; Smith et al. 2005). Interestingly, Schulte-Baukloh and colleagues demonstrated minimal post void residual volume by simultaneously injecting BoNT-A into the bladder and external urethral sphincter (Schulte-Baukloh et al. 2005a, b). Table 4.2 summarizes the noted incidence of idiopathic detrusor overactivity and neurogenic detrusor overactivity patients requiring clean intermittent catheterization following BoNT injection.

Although the efficacy of BoNT treatment has been demonstrated in all the studies currently cited, the impact of toxin dosage and delivery (i.e., toxin dose and dilution and the site and depth of injections) on the development of adverse events remains to be established. Kuo via multivariate analysis in 217 patients treated with onabotulinumtoxinA for IDO found that male gender and baseline post void residual urine volume >100 ml were independent predictors for acute urinary retention following treatment (Kuo et al. 2010). Sahai and colleagues evaluated the risk of the need for intermittent catheterization in 67 patients with IDO treated with 200 U of onabotulinumtoxinA (Sahai et al. 2009). They found that a projected isovolumetric pressure of less than or equal to 50 in women and a bladder contractility index of less than or equal to 120 in men predicted the need for intermittent catheterization.

> **Box 4.1: Phase 2B Clinical Trial Data of Onabotulinumtoxin A (Dmochowski et al. 2010)**
>
> Our personal experience with BoNT for OAB and IDO for over 10 years matches the Phase II study now bringing to a total four randomized placebo controlled clinical trials demonstrating the efficacy of onabotulinumtoxinA (Botox®, Allergan, Inc., Irvine, CA) in the treatment of refractory idiopathic overactive bladder (Anger et al. 2010; Dmochowski et al. 2010).
>
> Although not FDA approved, we believe there is an argument that BoNT may be considered as a standard treatment option for refractory OAB and IDO. Accepting BoNT as a standard treatment option for refractory OAB and IDO does not equate with recommending it as being first-line therapy. An Argument for recommending BoNT is that onabotulinumtoxinA treatment has been performed by many urologists and urogynecologists in a single office based setting with minimal morbidity. Mean duration of response averages 6–9 months and studies demonstrate similar efficacy with repeat treatments. An Argument against recommending BoNT is that BoNT treatment of overactive bladder carries the risk of an elevated post-void residual with the potential need for bladder catheterization.

4.5.1 Risk–Benefit Ratio

With OAB related costs estimated at over $12 billion US dollars annually (Hu et al. 2003), the health economic impact of each treatment modality must also be factored when considering the choice of therapy. One recent study determined that onabotulinumtoxinA was a cost effective treatment for urge urinary incontinence when

Table 4.2 Risk of clean intermittent catheterization after bladder botulinum toxin injection

Lead Author	Year	Condition	No. of pts treated with BoNT-A	Units of onabotulinumtoxinA injected	Trigone injected	Urethral sphincter injected	PVR (ml) criteria to start CIC	CIC (% of pts)
Rapp (Rapp et al. 2004)	2004	IDO	35	300	Yes	No	NA	0
Flynn (Flynn et al. 2004)	2004	IDO	7	150	No	No	NA	0
Werner (Werner et al. 2005)	2005	IDO	26	100	No	No	>100	8
Kuo (Kuo 2005)	2005	IDO	20	200	No	No	>250	30–50
Schulte-Baukloh (Schulte-Baukloh et al. 2005a)	2005	IDO	44	200–300	Yes	If pre-injection PVR >15 ml	NA (post-injection PVR <90 ml)	0
Schulte-Baukloh (Schulte-Baukloh et al. 2005b)	2005	IDO	7	300	Yes	Yes	NA (post-injection PVR <15 ml)	0
Schmid (Schmid et al. 2006)	2006	IDO	100	100	No	No	>400	4 (15/100 pts with PVR 150–200 ml)
Kuo (Kuo 2004)	2004	IDO+NDO	30	200	No	No	NA	20
Smith (Smith et al. 2005)	2005	IDO+NDO	42	100–300	Yes	No	NA (post-injection PVR 47 ml)	0
Popat (Popat et al. 2005)	2005	IDO+NDO	44	200–300	No	No	>100	69 (NDO) 19 (IDO)
Kessler (Kessler et al. 2005)	2005	IDO+NDO	22	300	No	No	>150	45 (NDO) 36 (IDO)

4.5 Side Effects

Study	Year	Type	N	Dose			PVR definition	CIC n (%)
Sahai (Sahai et al. 2007)	2007	IDO	16	200	No	No	>150	37.5
Brubaker (Brubaker et al. 2008)	2008	IDO	28	200	No	No	>200	43
Flynn (Flynn et al. 2009)	2009	IOAB	15	200–300	No	No	>100 + symptoms	7
Dmochowski (Dmochowski et al. 2010)	2010	IOAB	56	50	No	No	Not defined	5 (12.5% with PVR>200)
Dmochowski (Dmochowski et al. 2010)	2010	IOAB	55	100	No	No	Not defined	11 (14.5% with PVR>200)
Dmochowski (Dmochowski et al. 2010)	2010	IOAB	50	150	No	No	Not defined	20 (20% with PVR>200)
Dmochowski (Dmochowski et al. 2010)	2010	IOAB	52	200	No	No	Not defined	21 (28.8% with PVR>200)
Dmochowski (Dmochowski et al. 2010)	2010	IOAB	55	300	No	No	Not defined	16 (27.3% with PVR>200)

The main objective of this table is to demonstrate the risk defined by each author of clean intermittent catheterization (i.e., CIC) following bladder BoNT (onabotulinumtoxinA) injection in idiopathic (i.e., IDO) or mixed idiopathic and neurogenic (i.e., IDO + NDO) detrusor overactive patients. Post-void residual (PVR) data, unless otherwise stated, represent values determined by each investigator as warranting initiation of CIC. In many cases, these criteria or actual post-injection PVR data were not available and are represented by NA

compared to antimuscarinic therapy (Wu et al. 2009). A second study found that onabotulinumtoxinA bladder injection was cheaper than other treatment options such as sacral neuromodulation and augmentation cystoplasty, at least when considering initial costs and costs estimated over a 3 year period (Watanabe et al. 2010).

In the absence of data demonstrating a significantly greater clinical efficacy or cost benefit analysis, it seems unlikely that patients or clinicians will choose botulinum toxin as initial treatment of refractory OAB. Future studies should evaluate measures to optimize the risk-benefit ratio for botulinum toxin treatment. We recommend consideration of injection paradigms including trigone vs. non-trigone, dose dilution, depth of injection, and potential alternative delivery methods as (Chuang et al. 2009) avenues of research.

4.6 Conclusions

Overactive bladder is a common medical condition that can have a deleterious impact on a person's mental, physical, social, and financial well-being. Of those that are diagnosed and treated with front-line anticholinergic medications, a significant proportion of patients cease treatment due to lack of efficacy, cost of medications, or adverse side effects especially dry mouth and constipation. Although not approved by the regulatory agencies, recent data supports the use of botulinum toxin bladder injection as a viable therapeutic option in patients with refractory overactive bladder symptoms and idiopathic detrusor overactivity. We are excited at what the next 5 years will hold for this promising new therapy for the lower urinary tract.

References

Anger JT, Weinberg A, Suttorp MJ, Litwin MS, Shekelle PG (2010) Outcomes of intravesical botulinum toxin for idiopathic overactive bladder symptoms: a systematic review of the literature. J Urol 183(6):2258–2264

Apostolidis A, Dasgupta P, Denys P, Elneil S, Fowler CJ, Giannantoni A, Karsenty G, Schulte-Baukloh H, Schurch B, Wyndaele JJ (2009) Recommendations on the use of botulinum toxin in the treatment of lower urinary tract disorders and pelvic floor dysfunctions: a European consensus report. Eur Urol 55(1):100–119

Blasi J, Chapman ER, Link E, Binz T, Yamasaki S, De Camilli P, Sudhof TC, Niemann H, Jahn R (1993) Botulinum neurotoxin A selectively cleaves the synaptic protein SNAP-25. Nature 365(6442):160–163

Bosch JL (1998) Sacral neuromodulation in the treatment of the unstable bladder. Curr Opin Urol 8(4):287–291

Brubaker L, Richter HE, Visco A, Mahajan S, Nygaard I, Braun TM, Barber MD, Menefee S, Schaffer J, Weber AM, Wei J (2008) Refractory idiopathic urge urinary incontinence and botulinum A injection. J Urol 180(1):217–222

Chancellor MB, de Groat WC (1999) Intravesical capsaicin and resiniferatoxin therapy: spicing up the ways to treat the overactive bladder. J Urol 162(1):3–11

Chancellor MB, Fowler CJ, Apostolidis A, de Groat WC, Smith CP, Somogyi GT, Aoki KR (2008) Drug insight: biological effects of botulinum toxin A in the lower urinary tract. Nat Clin Pract Urol 5(6):319–328

References

Chuang YC, Tyagi P, Huang CC, Yoshimura N, Wu M, Kaufman J, Chancellor MB (2009) Urodynamic and immunohistochemical evaluation of intravesical botulinum toxin A delivery using liposomes. J Urol 182(2):786–792

Cohen BL, Caruso DJ, Kanagarajah P, Gousse AE (2009) Predictors of response to intradetrusor botulinum toxin-A injections in patients with idiopathic overactive bladder. Adv Urol 328364

Cui M, Khanijou S, Rubino J, Aoki KR (2004) Subcutaneous administration of botulinum toxin A reduces formalin-induced pain. Pain 107(1–2):125–133

Dmochowski R, Chapple C, Nitti VW, Chancellor M, Everaert K, Thompson C, Daniell G, Zhou J, Haag-Molkenteller C (2010) Efficacy and safety of onabotulinumtoxinA for idiopathic overactive bladder: a double-blind, placebo controlled, randomized, dose ranging trial. J Urol 184(6):2416–2422

Flynn MK, Webster GD, Amundsen CL (2004) The effect of botulinum-A toxin on patients with severe urge urinary incontinence. J Urol 172(6 Pt 1):2316–2320

Flynn MK, Amundsen CL, Perevich M, Liu F, Webster GD (2009) Outcome of a randomized, double-blind, placebo controlled trial of botulinum A toxin for refractory overactive bladder. J Urol 181(6):2608–2615

Hohenfellner M, Dahms SE, Matzel K, Thuroff JW (2000) Sacral neuromodulation for treatment of lower urinary tract dysfunction. BJU Int 85(suppl 3):10–19, discussion 22–13

Hu TW, Wagner TH, Bentkover JD, LeBlanc K, Piancentini A, Stewart WF, Corey R, Zhou SZ, Hunt TL (2003) Estimated economic costs of overactive bladder in the United States. Urology 61(6):1123–1128

Karsenty G, Elzayat E, Delapparent T, St-Denis B, Lemieux MC, Corcos J (2007) Botulinum toxin type A injections into the trigone to treat idiopathic overactive bladder do not induce vesicoureteral reflux. J Urol 177(3):1011–1014

Kessler TM, Danuser H, Schumacher M, Studer UE, Burkhard FC (2005) Botulinum A toxin injections into the detrusor: an effective treatment in idiopathic and neurogenic detrusor overactivity? Neurourol Urodyn 24(3):231–236

Kim HS, Hwang JH, Jeong ST, Lee YT, Lee PK, Suh YL, Shim JS (2003) Effect of muscle activity and botulinum toxin dilution volume on muscle paralysis. Dev Med Child Neurol 45(3):200–206

Kuo HC (2004) Urodynamic evidence of effectiveness of botulinum A toxin injection in treatment of detrusor overactivity refractory to anticholinergic agents. Urology 63(5):868–872

Kuo HC (2005) Clinical effects of suburothelial injection of botulinum A toxin on patients with nonneurogenic detrusor overactivity refractory to anticholinergics. Urology 66(1):94–98

Kuo HC (2007) Comparison of effectiveness of detrusor, suburothelial and bladder base injections of botulinum toxin a for idiopathic detrusor overactivity. J Urol 178(4 Pt 1):1359–1363

Kuo HC, Liao CH, Chung SD (2010) Adverse events of intravesical botulinum toxin A injections for idiopathic detrusor overactivity: risk factors and influence on treatment outcome. Eur Urol 58(6):919–926

Mehnert U, Boy S, Schmid M, Reitz A, von Hessling A, Hodler J, Schurch B (2009) A morphological evaluation of botulinum neurotoxin A injections into the detrusor muscle using magnetic resonance imaging. World J Urol 27(3):397–403

Meunier FA, Colasante C, Faille L, Gastard M, Molgo J (1996) Upregulation of calcitonin gene-related peptide at mouse motor nerve terminals poisoned with botulinum type-A toxin. Pflugers Arch 431(6 suppl 2):R297–R298

Popat R, Apostolidis A, Kalsi V, Gonzales G, Fowler CJ, Dasgupta P (2005) A comparison between the response of patients with idiopathic detrusor overactivity and neurogenic detrusor overactivity to the first intradetrusor injection of botulinum-A toxin. J Urol 174(3):984–989

Rapp DE, Lucioni A, Katz EE, O'Connor RC, Gerber GS, Bales GT (2004) Use of botulinum-A toxin for the treatment of refractory overactive bladder symptoms: an initial experience. Urology 63(6):1071–1075

Sahai A, Khan MS, Dasgupta P (2007) Efficacy of botulinum toxin-A for treating idiopathic detrusor overactivity: results from a single center, randomized, double-blind, placebo controlled trial. J Urol 177(6):2231–2236

Sahai A, Khan MS, Le Gall N, Dasgupta P (2008) Urodynamic assessment of poor responders after botulinum toxin-A treatment for overactive bladder. Urology 71(3):455–459

Sahai A, Sangster P, Kalsi V, Khan MS, Fowler CJ, Dasgupta P (2009) Assessment of urodynamic and detrusor contractility variables in patients with overactive bladder syndrome treated with botulinum toxin-A: is incomplete bladder emptying predictable? BJU Int 103(5):630–634

Schmid DM, Sauermann P, Werner M, Schuessler B, Blick N, Muentener M, Strebel RT, Perucchini D, Scheiner D, Schaer G, John H, Reitz A, Hauri D, Schurch B (2006) Experience with 100 cases treated with botulinum-A toxin injections in the detrusor muscle for idiopathic overactive bladder syndrome refractory to anticholinergics. J Urol 176(1):177–185

Schulte-Baukloh H, Weiss C, Stolze T, Herholz J, Sturzebecher B, Miller K, Knispel HH (2005a) Botulinum-A toxin detrusor and sphincter injection in treatment of overactive bladder syndrome: objective outcome and patient satisfaction. Eur Urol 48(6):984–990, discussion 990

Schulte-Baukloh H, Weiss C, Stolze T, Sturzebecher B, Knispel HH (2005b) Botulinum-A toxin for treatment of overactive bladder without detrusor overactivity: urodynamic outcome and patient satisfaction. Urology 66(1):82–87

Smith CP, Chancellor MB (2004) Emerging role of botulinum toxin in the management of voiding dysfunction. J Urol 171(6 Pt 1):2128–2137

Smith CP, Chancellor MB (2005) Simplified bladder botulinum-toxin delivery technique using flexible cystoscope and 10 sites of injection. J Endourol 19(7):880–882

Smith CP, Nishiguchi J, O'Leary M, Yoshimura N, Chancellor MB (2005) Single-institution experience in 110 patients with botulinum toxin A injection into bladder or urethra. Urology 65(1):37–41

Stewart WF, Van Rooyen JB, Cundiff GW, Abrams P, Herzog AR, Corey R, Hunt TL, Wein AJ (2003) Prevalence and burden of overactive bladder in the United States. World J Urol 20(6):327–336

Van Kerrebroeck EV, van der Aa HE, Bosch JL, Koldewijn EL, Vorsteveld JH, Debruyne FM (1997) Sacral rhizotomies and electrical bladder stimulation in spinal cord injury. Part I: clinical and urodynamic analysis. Dutch Study Group on Sacral Anterior Root Stimulation. Eur Urol 31(3):263–271

Watanabe JH, Campbell JD, Ravelo A, Chancellor MB, Kowalski J, Sullivan SD (2010) Cost analysis of interventions for antimuscarinic refractory patients with overactive bladder. Urology 76(4):835–840

Welch MJ, Purkiss JR, Foster KA (2000) Sensitivity of embryonic rat dorsal root ganglia neurons to *Clostridium botulinum* neurotoxins. Toxicon 38(2):245–258

Werner M, Schmid DM, Schussler B (2005) Efficacy of botulinum-A toxin in the treatment of detrusor overactivity incontinence: a prospective nonrandomized study. Am J Obstet Gynecol 192(5):1735–1740

Wu JM, Siddiqui NY, Amundsen CL, Myers ER, Havrilesky LJ, Visco AG (2009) Cost-effectiveness of botulinum toxin a versus anticholinergic medications for idiopathic urge incontinence. J Urol 181(5):2181–2186

BoNT for Bladder and Pelvic Pain

5.1 Introduction

Botulinum toxin (BoNT) has demonstrated effectiveness in the treatment of several pain disorders including focal dystonia, cervical dystonia/spastic torticollis, spasmodic dysphonia, oromandibular dystonia, temporomandibular disorder, refractory myofascial pain syndrome, and tension- and migraine-type headache (Smith et al. 2002). These positive results of BoNT helping pain stimulated interest on the use of BoNT for a variety of genitourinary pain conditions. BoNT's mechanism of action for pain relief is thought to be primarily based on eliminating tonic muscle contraction and, subsequently, blunting nociceptive responses. In addition, BoNT has been shown to inhibit central glutamate release, thus diminishing excitatory amino acid receptors important to the central windup process and pain perception (Smith et al. 2002). Central desensitization may be indirectly mediated via peripheral desensitization resulting from BoNT-induced inhibition of neurotransmitter release from primary sensory neurons (Aoki 2005; Chuang et al. 2004).

5.2 Indications

Interstitial cystitis/Bladder Pain Syndrome (IC/PBS) is a syndrome of chronic lower urinary tract irritative symptoms and pelvic pain in the absence of other pathology. Interstitial cystitis and painful bladder syndrome may be descriptions of the same entity, distinct from other pelvic/genitourinary pain syndromes (Bogart et al. 2007; Nickel 2004). However, in many patients bladder pain is just one component of a more diffuse pelvic pain syndrome that may also include pain in the pelvic floor, urethral sphincters, vulva, or prostate.

While traditionally viewed to be more common in women, the syndrome affects both men and women; the incidence in men may be underestimated as some men with IC/PBS may be misclassified as having chronic prostatis/male chronic pelvic pain syndrome (Forrest et al. 2007). Pain and urinary frequency in the absence of other identifiable cause are consistent characteristics of the syndrome (Fig. 5.1) (Hanno

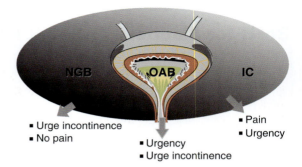

Fig. 5.1 Diagram depicting spectrum of voiding dysfunction from conditions associated with primarily motor abnormality (neurogenic bladder dysfunction (*NGB*)) to those primarily associated with a sensory nerve disorder (interstitial cystitis (*IC*))

et al. 1999; Nickel 2004). The pain typically increases with bladder filling, is usually suprapubic but may localize elsewhere in the pelvis and perineum, and is often extreme in intensity especially during flare-ups. In practical clinical terms, the diagnosis is made by a combination of a history of urgency/frequency, bladder pain in the absence of infection or malignancy, and typical examination findings of tenderness.

A symptom questionnaire may be helpful, such as the University of Wisconsin Interstitial Cystitis Scale, the O'Leary-Sant Symptom Index, or the Pelvic Pain and Urinary Frequency Score (Evans and Sant 2007). The cystoscopic presence of glomerulations after hydrodistension, long-accepted as diagnostic of IC/PBS, has not been proven (Fall et al. 2004). Standard treatments include oral and intravesical agents, bladder hydrodistension, as well as adjusting external factors such as diet and stress that might be exacerbating a patient's symptoms. If a patient is refractory to these treatments, BoNT injection should be offered as a therapeutic option.

5.3 What Is the Work-Up

5.3.1 History and Physical Examination

One should do a complete history including symptoms related to onset and trigger of pain. Past medical history should include possible history of abuse and any other incidents that may have triggered the wind up of pain. Response to any medications or intravesical therapies, especially if they have had BoNT in the past should be elicited. Urogenital issues including sexual history, bladder diary, and irritable bowel syndrome, or constipation should also be assessed. Physical exam should include a bimanual pelvic exam in females and digital rectal exam in males in order to identify trigger points that will reproduce or exacerbate a patient's pain symptoms.

5.3.2 Urodynamic Evaluation

We do not routinely perform urodynamic testing for every patient with pain but we respect experts who feel urodynamic testing is important in ruling out lower urinary tract diseases that may present with pain. We do feel it is helpful in cases of dysfunctional micturition to rule out potential anatomic obstruction at the level of the bladder neck, prostate, external sphincter or post-female sling and pelvic prolapse repair.

Electromyography can be performed concurrently to diagnose detrusor sphincter dyssynergia but patch electrodes are preferred (e.g., needle electrodes are uncomfortable for most sensate individuals). When combined with fluoroscopy, additional data on the mechanics, anatomy, and structure of the bladder, urethra, and the presence of vesicoureteral reflux can be obtained in real time.

5.4 How to Do It

5.4.1 Patient Preparation

Similar issues arise for injection for the treatment of pain as for neurogenic and idiopathic overactive bladder. Some key issues for pain indication to consider are listed below. Procedures, guidelines, and rules may differ slightly amongst various centers and countries.

- Urine analysis should be negative at the time of the procedure (if the patient has a history of chronic bacteriuria, appropriate preoperative antibiotic coverage is indicated).
- Since the incidence of pelvic pain is more common in younger women, attention for potential pregnancy and birth control is encouraged.
- Since the patient has bothersome pain and may be on significant analgesics already, a plan on peri- and post-procedure pain control should be discussed and agreed upon prior to BoNT injection.
- Risk of retention and potential for intermittent self- catheterization.
- Informed consent with notation of off-label use and drug warning
- Sterile cystoscopic preparation with standard antibiotic coverage for a minor cystoscopic procedure
- Use of urethral and bladder local anesthesia is helpful and general anesthesia may need to be considered in selective patients.

Once again, the risk of incomplete emptying and retention is especially important in patients with pain. The clinician in a compassionate attempt to help a patient with severe pain and decreased quality of life would not want retention and induce worse pain with intermittent or indwelling catheterization. The patient should be aware, give consent and be able to perform catheterization to avoid a treatment that turns out to be worse than the problem it intends to treat.

5.4.2 Cystoscope

Both rigid and flexible cystoscopic techniques work well in our hands and those of most experts without an apparent difference in clinical outcomes. Physician preference and institutional practice usually decide what technique is used. We believe in focusing on the use of an adequate amount and duration of contact of lidocaine before injecting.

Flexible scope: We use flexible cystoscopy in the office for the majority of cases to minimize cost to patients if they are paying the procedure out of pocket. The flexible scope accommodates a 27 Fr flexible Olympus® injection needle (disposable) which must be passed through a reusable sheath. Office procedures with only local anesthesia are adequate for most of our patients. Patients appreciate the convenience of an office procedure.

Rigid scope: While any rigid cystoscope will work, one author (CPS) prefers using an ACMI® Cystoscope with 12° lens, bridged with an accessory working element loaded with a 25 gauge Cook® Williams Needle. The rigid scope allows for easier orientation within the bladder compared to a flexible cystoscope, the working element facilitates rapid injection into the bladder, and the 25 gauge needle minimizes bleeding and potential backflow from the injection sites. Urethral and pelvic floor injections, if done concomitantly, can easily be accomplished with use of a 22 gauge short spinal needle (i.e., urethral sphincter injections) and a disposable pudendal nerve block kit (i.e., levator muscle injections) (Fig. 5.2).

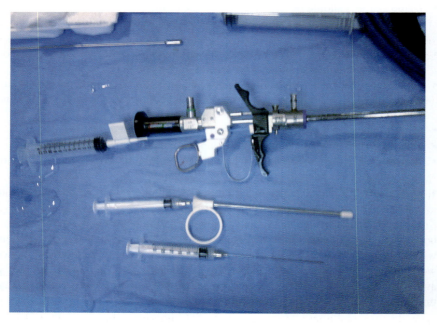

Fig. 5.2 Photograph depicting equipment used to inject BoNT in the case study. *Top* of photograph shows ACMI® Cystoscope with 12° lens, bridged with an Accessory Working Element and loaded with a 25 gauge Cook® Williams Needle. This setup allows for easy orientation within the bladder, rapid injection requiring only one individual, and minimal bleeding or risk of backflow of toxin. The *middle* of the photograph depicts the needle/trocar equipment from a disposable pudendal nerve block kit that is useful to localize and inject the levator muscles transvaginally. The *bottom* of photograph displays the 22 gauge short spinal needle used to target the external urethral sphincter and vulvar areas

The bladder volume is typically kept at 100–200 ml keeping in mind what is the functional bladder capacity of the patients. The first observable change noted by patients following BoNT injection is a reduction in urgency and frequency after 4–7 days. These variables continue to improve significantly by 4 weeks. Pelvic pain intimately associated with bladder filling or emptying should also improve with concomitant reductions in frequency and urgency.

If general anesthesia is utilized, we always combine onabotulinumtoxinA injection with a hydrodistension and intravesical instillation. In fact, literature demonstrates that hydrodistension can enhance the effect of bladder onabotulinumtoxinA injection (Liu and Kuo 2007).

5.4.3 Botulinum Toxin Reconstitution

Each vial of 100 U onabotulinumtoxinA is usually reconstituted to 10 ml with injectable preservative-free saline, making the concentration equivalent to 10 U/ml. OnabotulinumtoxinA is kept in the refrigerator according to instruction and we usually do not reconstitute the onabotulinumtoxinA until we know that infection has been ruled out or an appropriate antibiotic started to avoid wastage.

Each vial of abobotulinumtoxinA contains either 300 U (i.e., for glabellar lines) or 500 U (i.e., for cervical dystonia). Studies have documented dilutions with preservative-free saline to a concentration of 25–100 U/ml.

Each vial of rimabotulinumtoxinB contains 5,000 U/ml and is already reconstituted. Although few studies have used onabotulinumtoxinA to treat bladder overactivity, most have diluted to a concentration of 250 U/ml.

5.4.4 Dose

We routinely use 100 U of onabotulinumtoxinA for first time bladder injection in the majority of our IC/PBS patients. Based on the experience of others and ourselves, we generally have not found a benefit in increasing bladder injection dosage above 100 U in patients who do not respond at all to the initial treatment (Liu and Kuo 2007). In particular, we are concerned that the higher dosage would cause urinary retention, an intolerable de novo complaint in this patient population. However, in select patients with marginal improvement to 100 U of onabotulinumtoxinA and in those willing to accept the risk of intermittent catheterization, 200 U of onabotulinumtoxinA has been utilized with some success. Typical doses in adult patients treated with abobotulinumtoxinA is 300–500 U, and for rimabotulinumtoxinB doses range between 2,500–5,000 U.

The potency units of all commercially available BoNT's are specific to that particular preparation and assay method utilized. They are not interchangeable with other preparations of BoNT products and, therefore, units of biological activity of one toxin preparation cannot be compared or converted into units of any other botulinum toxins products assessed with any other specific assay method.

5.4.5 Depth, Location, and Amount of Injection

We usually inject 1 ml/site (10 U onabotulinumtoxinA/ml) so, for example, if we are using 100 U there will be approximately ten injection sites (i.e., dissolving each bottle in 10 ml of preservative-free saline).

5.4.6 Injection Technique

How deep should BoNT be injected into the bladder? Recent studies of BoNT injection for overactive bladder and idiopathic detrusor overactivity have used suburothelial delivery to potentially target the suburothelial sensory pathway rather than paralysis of detrusor muscle in the treatment of the overactive bladder (Kuo 2006). In many neurogenic detrusor overactive patients who are already catheterizing and where complete paralysis is the treatment objective, perhaps deeper detrusor injections should be the approach used. Unfortunately, especially in IC/PBS bladders with a thin bladder wall, it might be difficult to differentiate suburothelium from detrusor muscle.

In our experience, the avoidance of retention is paramount in IC/PBS and therefore we continue to prefer superficial suburothelial depth of injection in IC/PBS patients.

5.4.6.1 Trigone Injection

A successful outcome was reported with BoNT injection into only the trigone and bladder base (Smith and Chancellor 2005). The rationale for trigone injection is that this portion of the urinary bladder contains a prominent parasympathetic plexus of BoNT receptor-positive nerves, although the role of this plexus on bladder urgency sensation and DO has not been fully explored (Coelho et al. 2010). This also does not take into account a possible therapeutic effect of BoNT on the abundant sensory nerves within the trigone. Although vesical urleteral reflux might be a potential complication after BoNT in these areas, studies have not supported this claim (Karsenty et al. 2007; Mascarenhas et al. 2008). In the present authors' personal experience over the past 10 years, submucosal trigone and bladder base injections of BoNT are associated with a low incidence of urinary retention and a similar efficacy to intradetrusor injection.

It should be emphasized that no standardized injection technique exists for BoNT injection in lower urinary tract tissues. Different bladder injection paradigms have been described (i.e., trigone vs. trigone-sparing) although none has been proven to be superior to the other.

5.4.6.2 Combined Bladder and Urethral/Prostate/Levator Injections

In our experience, many women with IC/PBS also have pelvic floor pain as well. Symptoms include pain in urethra, and dyspareunia. Treatment of these patients also includes injection of the urethral sphincter, levator muscles, and vulvar areas (See Chap. 7 on Sphincter injections for directions on sphincter and levator injections in females). Thus, female patients may be injected with up to 300–400 U of onabotulinumtoxinA in one setting with 100 U in bladder, 50–66 U in urethral sphincter, 33–50 U in vulva posterior fourchette and 100–200 U in levator muscles.

In men, as in women, physical exam is useful to identify the trigger points of their pain symptoms. Targeting of the prostate or rhabdosphincter in males with bladder and pelvic floor symptoms is based on elicitation of pain with palpation of these areas on digital rectal exam (See chapters on Prostate and Sphincter injections). If combined with bladder injections, we typically inject 100 U in the bladder trigone and 100–200 U in the prostate or external urethral sphincter transurethrally using a 27 gauge Olympus endoscopic needle with sheath.

5.4.7 Post-procedure and Follow-Up

We instruct our patient's that they may notice some pain and blood-tinged urine, as well as possible difficulty urinating following treatment. These symptoms should resolve within 24 h and they should call and contact us immediately if they have any questions or concerns. We discuss the appropriate antibiotic coverage and risk of infection in these patients who often have more bladder infections. For those who are not already on intermittent catheterization, we formulate a plan if urinary retention occurs.

We always remind the patients that it takes several days to notice a gradual improvement in symptoms. Similarly, it generally takes several days for a patient to notice impaired voiding and we would instruct that patient to start self-catheterization if clinically necessary.

5.4.8 How Long Does It Last and When Is Botulinum Toxin Injection Repeated

It generally takes about 1 week for our patients to notice some relief of symptoms. If the injection helps, he or she will gain further improvement that usually reaches a maximal benefit at about 1 month. The beneficial effect is usually maintained for 4–6 months in IC/PBS and pelvic pain patients. Subsequently, urinary frequency/urgency and bladder/pelvic pain symptoms reoccur. These are signals we tell our patients to look for and to contact us to schedule a repeat injection.

5.5 What Are the Results

5.5.1 Clinical Results IC/PBS

The first report was a case series of 13 women with National Institute of Health-defined IC/PBS (Smith et al. 2004). The patients underwent submucosal transure-

Case Study 5.1: A 34-year-old woman with IC/CPPS
Chief Complaint: frequency, urgency, suprapubic pain, and dyspareunia

Presentation: A 34-year-old woman was referred by a local urologist with a recent diagnosis of interstitial cystitis after having been treated for "recurrent urinary tract infections" for 7 years. She has previously been evaluated by a gynecologist via pelvic u/s and diagnostic laparoscopy with no evidence of endometriosis or other uterine/ovarian pathology. The patient has tried multiple oral and intravesical treatments for her symptoms in addition to dietary and social adjustments without lasting improvement. She also tried acupuncture and tibial nerve stimulation without success. She is home-bound on most days and bedridden during severe flare-ups. She was recently married and desires a family but her symptoms prevent her from engaging in sexual activity. She comes to your office stating "please remove my bladder."

Physical exam revealed suprapubic tenderness to mild-moderate palpation. On pelvic exam, the patient demonstrated exquisite tenderness on palpation of her levator muscles, bilaterally and with bladder base palpation. The patient's pelvic floor muscles were tonically active but she could only elicit a weak kegel upon command. Patient had a previous cystogram demonstrating a relatively smooth walled bladder with adequate capacity and no vesicoureteral reflux (Fig. 5.3).

The patient was counseled about the risks of cystectomy and the significant potential for persistent pelvic pain. She was offered other minimally invasive options including BoNT injection and sacral neuromodulation. The patient desired to undergo BoNT injection of the bladder, urethra, vulva, and pelvic floor. She declined sacral neuromodulation because of desire to start a family and her slender body build Due to the patient's severe pain symptoms, the procedure was performed under general anesthesia in conjunction with a hydrodistension ad intravesical instillation of drugs.

Treatment: After informed consent, the patient underwent cystoscopy with hydrodistension, onabotulinumtoxinA injection to the bladder trigone and base in ten sites (100 U/10 ml) followed by intravesical instillation of a drug cocktail. A second vial of 100 U of onabotulinumtoxinA was diluted in 3 ml of preservative free saline. Using a 22-gauge short spinal needle, 1 ml (i.e., 33 U) was injected onto each side of the external urethral sphincter by inserting the needle for 1.5 cm at the 3 o'clock and 9 o'clock within the periurethral folds. The remaining 1 ml divided into 0.5 ml aliquots and was injected into the 5 and 7 o'clock positions in the posterior fourchette. A final vial of onabotulinumtoxinA was diluted in 3 ml of preservative-free saline. Using a disposable pudendal nerve block kit, a total of four injections were made targeting the pubococcygeus and puborectalis muscles on either side.

Outcome: Within 1 week, the patient noticed a significant decrease in pelvic floor spasms followed by a progressive decrease in frequency and urgency. Concomitant with the reduction in frequency/urgency and pelvic spasms was a marked reduction in pain. The patient was able to reduce her pain med requirements by 50%. In addition, she was able to engage in sexual activity with only mild and transient discomfort afterward. If her symptoms continue to be stabilized with onabotulinumtoxinA, the patient plans on trying to time her pregnancy for shortly after her next injection cycle.

Fig. 5.3 Cystogram demonstrating a bladder of over 300 ml capacity, closed bladder neck, no vesicoureteral reflux and no trabeculation

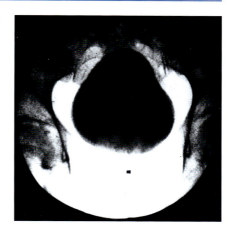

Fig. 5.4 Interstitial cystitis symptom index (*ICSI*) and interstitial cystitis problem index (*ICPI*) scores before and after onabotulinumtoxinA treatment. Following onabotulinumtoxinA treatment, mean ICSI scores decreased from 17.0 ± 1.9 to 5.3 ± 0.4 ($*p<0.05$), and mean ICPI scores reduced from 15.7 ± 0.4 to 4.5 ± 2.5 ($\#p<0.05$) (Reprint permission required Smith et al. 2004)

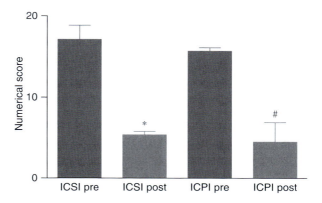

thral injections of 100–200 U of abobotulinumtoxinA (seven patients) or onabotulinumtoxinA (six patients) into 20–30 sites in the trigone and bladder base. Validated questionnaire (Interstitial Cystitis Symptom Index, Interstitial Cystitis Problem Index) or voiding charts and a visual analog pain scale were evaluated at baseline, 1 month and subsequently at 3 month intervals. Statistically significant improvements in frequency, nocturia and pain were observed 1 month following treatment, in addition to improvements in first desire to void and cystometric capacity in those patients so evaluated (Figs. 5.4 and 5.5). Onset of symptom relief was 5–7 days following treatment, and mean duration of symptom relief was 3.7 months.

Giannantoni and colleagues were among the first to report on the effects of onabotulinumtoxinA for IC/PBS: A pilot study of 12 women and 2 men were reported (Giannantoni et al. 2006). Under short general anesthesia, patients were given injections of 200 U of commercially available onabotulinumtoxinA submucosally in the trigone and bladder floor under cystoscopic control. Overall, 12 patients (85.7%) reported subjective improvement at 1 and 3 months follow-up. The

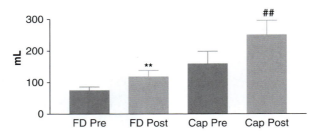

Fig. 5.5 Urodynamic parameters before and after abobotulinumtoxinA treatment. Significant increases in first desire to void (e.g., FD) (74.6 ± 11.8 ml to 118 ± 20.4 ml, $*p<0.01$) and maximum bladder capacity (e.g., Cap) (159 ± 39.9 ml to 250 ± 46.10 ml, $\#p<0.01$) were observed following treatment (Copyright obtained Smith et al. 2004)

mean visual analogue pain score was significantly reduced at 1 and 3 months after treatment and daytime and nighttime urinary frequency decreased. Two patients reported incomplete bladder emptying.

Giannantoni and associates more recently reported on the 2 year efficacy and tolerability of onabotulinumtoxinA injections in IC/PBS patients (Giannantoni et al. 2010). Thirteen women were prospectively included in the study. A total of 58 injections were administered in 13 women with IC/PBS with a mean of 4.8 injections/patient and a mean duration of 5.25 months between injections. Two hundred units of onabotulinumtoxinA were used in all patients. At 1 and 4 month follow-up, ten patients reported a subjective improvement in their symptoms. Mean VAS scores, and mean daytime and night-time urinary frequency decreased significantly. Nine patients at 1 month and seven at the 4-month check-up complained of dysuria. The three non-responders to the first intravesical treatment session underwent another treatment 3 months later with satisfactory results. Beneficial effects persisted in all patients at 1 and 2 year follow-up.

Somewhat less encouraging is a case series of 8 women and 2 men with chronic IC/PBS unresponsive to other therapy (Kuo 2005). Five patients were injected suburothelially with 100 U of onabotulinumtoxinA (20 sites), while the other five patients had an additional 100 U of onabotulinumtoxinA injected into the trigone. While functional and cystometric bladder capacity increased and frequency and pain scores improved mildly, significant improvements were noted in only two patients. No patient was symptom-free following treatment with BoNT. In addition, there were no therapeutic or adverse differences between the non-trigone and trigone injection groups.

In a recent study, Liu and Kuo compared the therapeutic results of intravesical onabotulinumtoxinA of 100 U or 200 U plus hydrodistention and hydrodistention alone (2007). Sixty-seven patients with IC/PBS who had failed conventional treatments were enrolled. Forty-four patients received suburothelial injection with 200 U ($n=15$) or 100 U ($n=29$) of onabotulinumtoxinA followed by cystoscopic hydrodistention 2 weeks later (BoNT group). Control group (23 patients) received identical hydrodistention procedure without onabotulinumtoxinA injection. The symptom score decreased in all three groups, but pain scale reduction, functional bladder capacity, and cystometric bladder capacity increased only in the onabotulinumtoxinA groups at 3 months. Among 44 patients in the onabotulinumtoxinA group, 31 (70.5%) had a successful result at 6 months, compared to only in 8 (34.8%) patients treated with hydrodistention alone ($P<0.001$).

Liu and Kuo's study demonstrated that intravesical injections of BoNT plus hydrodistention increased bladder capacity and provided long-term pain relief in patients with IC/PBS and that these effects were superior to those obtained with hydrodistention alone. Increasing the dose of onabotulinumtoxinA from 100 to 200 U, however, did not provide an additive benefit in terms of pain relief or bladder capacity increase. By contrast, the higher dose of onabotulinumtoxinA was associated with increased incidence of difficult urination and urinary retention.

Tirumuru and associates (2010) report a recent systemic review of randomized controlled trials and prospective studies of relevance of BoNT for IC/PBS. Ten (three randomized controlled trials and seven prospective cohort) studies with a total of 260 participants were included. Eight studies reported improvement in symptoms. Urodynamic parameters were variable and meta-analysis was not performed due to heterogeneity in outcomes reporting. Of the 260 patients, 19 needed to self-catheterize at some point after BoNT injection. The authors noted that current evidence suggests a trend towards short-term benefit for IC/PSB patients with bladder BoNT injections but further studies are needed.

5.5.2 Chronic Female Pelvic Pain Syndromes

A recent case series reported 24 women with significant vaginismus for whom standard therapies had failed (Ghazizadeh and Nikzad 2004). The mean age in this study was 25 years, and all were premenopausal. At a mean of 12.4 months follow-up, after onabotulinumtoxinA injection with 150–400 U 9.6% were found to have little to no muscular resistance at examination, and 75% had achieved successful intercourse. There were no recurrences, nor were there any significant side effects noted. A pilot study of onabotulinumtoxinA injection of pubococcygeus and puborectalis for the treatment of chronic pelvic pain in 12 women with chronic pelvic pain and pelvic floor muscle hypertonicity demonstrated improvements in hypertonicity and symptoms (Jarvis et al. 2004). Forty units of onabotulinumtoxinA were injected transvaginally into the puborectalis and pubococcygeus muscles bilaterally in a total of four sites, using three different concentrations of onabotulinumtoxinA (10, 20, and 100 U/ml). At 12 weeks follow-up, significant reduction in pain scores for dyspareunia and dysmenorrhea, and improvements in sexual activity and bladder function scores were observed.

In contrast, a double blind randomized clinical trial of BoNT versus saline in 60 patients with 2 years or more of chronic pelvic pain demonstrated no subjective difference between treatments (Abbott et al. 2006). Patients received either onabotulinumtoxinA 80 U (20 U/ml) or normal saline injections into the puborectalis and pubococcygeus muscles. After 26 weeks of follow-up, quality of life measures were improved in both onabotulinumtoxinA and placebo groups without statistical significance between the groups. However, objective reductions in pelvic floor pressure were observed in the onabotulinumtoxinA group compared to placebo.

5.5.3 Chronic Prostatis/Male Chronic Pelvic Pain Syndrome (CP/CPPS)

Only one clinical study specifically addressed the use of BoNT for the treatment of CP/CPPS (Zermann et al. 2000). Eleven men with chronic prostatic pain of greater than 12 months duration, age 32–66 years old were studied. OnabotulinumtoxinA (i.e., 200 units) was administered by transurethral perisphincteric injection under direct vision using a 22 gauge Bard needle via three to four injection sites. At 2–4 week follow-up, 9 of 11 patients reported subjective improvement. Visual pain analogue scores decreased from 7.2 to 1.6. In addition, significant decreases in pelvic floor tenderness, functional urethral length, urethral closure pressure, post void residual urine volume, and increases in average and maximal uroflow rate were observed. One patient developed stress urinary incontinence; however, no other problems were noted.

5.5.4 Radiation and Inflammatory Cystitis

Radiation cystitis is a severe but rare late complication of pelvic radiotherapy. Symptoms include urinary frequency, and urgency based on impairment of storage function of the organ. Similarly, intravesical BCG therapy for superficial bladder cancer often induces BCG cystitis and compromises bladder storage function. The BCG cystitis typically consists of an acute inflammation of the bladder wall in conjunction with the formation of granulomas (Palou et al. 2001).

Symptomatic treatment of radiation cystitis and BCG cystitis is challenging to the clinicians. Chuang and colleagues reported the clinical use of BoNT to patients with radiation and BCG induced cystitis (Chuang et al. 2008). Following bladder injection with 100–200 U of onabotulinumtoxinA, 7 out of 8 symptomatic patients demonstrated significant improvement (Figs. 5.6 and 5.7). No adverse event occurred after bladder onabotulinumtoxinA injection in these challenging patients. The potential benefit of bladder BoNT injection for refractory radiation and BCG

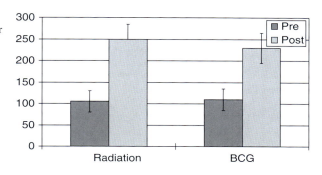

Fig. 5.6 Change in bladder capacity (*ml*) before and after BoNT in radiation and BCG inflammatory cystitis (Copyright obtained Chuang et al. 2008)

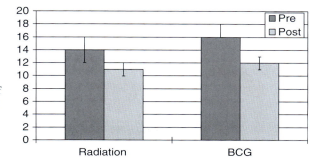

Fig. 5.7 Change in 24 h urinary frequency (number of micturitions/24 h) before and after BoNT in radiation and BCG inflammatory cystitis (Copyright obtained Chuang et al. 2008)

cystitis given these early results is encouraging. However, these results are based on a small case series and formal clinical trials should be undertaken to fully address a role for BoNT treatment of these refractory conditions.

5.6　Conclusions

The use of botulinum toxin in the treatment of chronic genitourinary pain syndromes holds promise. The toxin likely provides relief by means of a combination of chemical denervation of striated muscle, thereby relieving muscle tension and its induced pain, as well as direct anti-nociceptive effects. The latter may be the prominent mechanism of relief in interstitial cystitis/painful bladder syndrome (Fig. 5.8). Acceptance of a descriptive taxonomy of pelvic pain syndromes should precede prospective randomized trials with standardized outcome measures, in order to fully evaluate the clinical effectiveness of this treatment modality. Continuing efforts toward understanding the anti-nociceptive actions of botulinum toxin will more clearly define its role in specific pain syndromes.

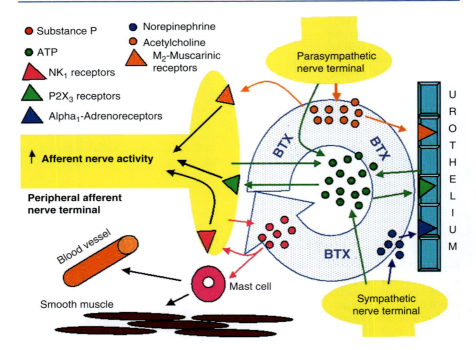

Fig. 5.8 Schematic diagram depicting neuronal (parasympathetic and sympathetic) and non-neuronal (e.g., urothelium) sources of various neurotransmitters (e.g., ATP, acetylcholine, norepinephrine, and substance P) that interact in a circuitous fashion to modulate bladder afferent nerve activity. *Circular arrow* depicts sites of action where botulinum toxin (*BTX*) may inhibit neurotransmitter release, reduce sensory nerve excitability and, thus, decrease clinical symptoms of urinary frequency, urgency, and pain (Copyright obtained Smith et al. 2004)

References

Abbott JA, Jarvis SK, Lyons SD, Thomson A, Vancaille TG (2006) Botulinum toxin type A for chronic pain and pelvic floor spasm in women: a randomized controlled trial. Obstet Gynecol 108(4):915–923

Aoki KR (2005) Review of a proposed mechanism for the antinociceptive action of botulinum toxin type A. Neurotoxicology 26(5):785–793

Bogart LM, Berry SH, Clemens JQ (2007) Symptoms of interstitial cystitis, painful bladder syndrome and similar diseases in women: a systematic review. J Urol 177(2):450–456

Chuang YC, Yoshimura N, Huang CC, Chiang PH, Chancellor MB (2004) Intravesical botulinum toxin a administration produces analgesia against acetic acid induced bladder pain responses in rats. J Urol 172(4 Pt 1):1529–1532

Chuang YC, Kim DK, Chiang PH, Chancellor MB (2008) Bladder botulinum toxin A injection can benefit patients with radiation and chemical cystitis. BJU Int 102(6):704–706

Coelho A, Dinis P, Pinto R, Gorgal T, Silva C, Silva A, Silva J, Cruz CD, Cruz F, Avelino A (2010) Distribution of the high-affinity binding site and intracellular target of botulinum toxin type A in the human bladder. Eur Urol 57(5):884–890

References

Evans RJ, Sant GR (2007) Current diagnosis of interstitial cystitis: an evolving paradigm. Urology 69(4 suppl):S64–S72

Fall M, Baranowski AP, Fowler CJ, Lepinard V, Malone-Lee JG, Messelink EJ, Oberpenning F, Osborne JL, Schumacher S (2004) EAU guidelines on chronic pelvic pain. Eur Urol 46(6):681–689

Forrest JB, Nickel JC, Moldwin RM (2007) Chronic prostatitis/chronic pelvic pain syndrome and male interstitial cystitis: enigmas and opportunities. Urology 69(4 suppl):S60–S63

Ghazizadeh S, Nikzad M (2004) Botulinum toxin in the treatment of refractory vaginismus. Obstet Gynecol 104(5 Pt 1):922–925

Giannantoni A, Costantini E, Di Stasi SM, Tascini MC, Bini V, Porena M (2006) Botulinum A toxin intravesical injections in the treatment of painful bladder syndrome: a pilot study. Eur Urol 49(4):704–709

Giannantoni A, Mearini E, Del Zingaro M, Proietti S, Porena M (2010) Two-year efficacy and safety of botulinum a toxin intravesical injections in patients affected by refractory painful bladder syndrome. Curr Drug Deliv 7(1):1–4

Hanno PM, Landis JR, Matthews-Cook Y, Kusek J, Nyberg L Jr (1999) The diagnosis of interstitial cystitis revisited: lessons learned from the National Institutes of Health Interstitial Cystitis Database study. J Urol 161(2):553–557

Jarvis SK, Abbott JA, Lenart MB, Steensma A, Vancaillie TG (2004) Pilot study of botulinum toxin type A in the treatment of chronic pelvic pain associated with spasm of the levator ani muscles. Aust N Z J Obstet Gynaecol 44(1):46–50

Karsenty G, Elzayat E, Delapparent T, St-Denis B, Lemieux MC, Corcos J (2007) Botulinum toxin type a injections into the trigone to treat idiopathic overactive bladder do not induce vesicoureteral reflux. J Urol 177(3):1011–1014

Kuo HC (2005) Preliminary results of suburothelial injection of botulinum a toxin in the treatment of chronic interstitial cystitis. Urol Int 75(2):170–174

Kuo HC (2006) Will suburothelial injection of small dose of botulinum A toxin have similar therapeutic effects and less adverse events for refractory detrusor overactivity? Urology 68(5):993–997; discussion 997–998

Liu HT, Kuo HC (2007) Intravesical botulinum toxin A injections plus hydrodistension can reduce nerve growth factor production and control bladder pain in interstitial cystitis. Urology 70(3):463–468

Mascarenhas F, Cocuzza M, Gomes CM, Leao N (2008) Trigonal injection of botulinum toxin-A does not cause vesicoureteral reflux in neurogenic patients. Neurourol Urodyn 27(4):311–314

Nickel JC (2004) Interstitial cystitis: the paradigm shifts: international consultations on interstitial cystitis. Rev Urol 6(4):200–202

Palou J, Rodriguez-Villamil L, Andreu-Crespo A, Salvador-Bayarri J, Vicente-Rodriguez J (2001) Intravesical treatment of severe bacillus Calmette-Guerin cystitis. Int Urol Nephrol 33(3):485–489

Smith CP, Chancellor MB (2005) Simplified bladder botulinum-toxin delivery technique using flexible cystoscope and 10 sites of injection. J Endourol 19(7):880–882

Smith HS, Audette J, Royal MA (2002) Botulinum toxin in pain management of soft tissue syndromes. Clin J Pain 18(6 suppl):S147–S154

Smith CP, Radziszewski P, Borkowski A, Somogyi GT, Boone TB, Chancellor MB (2004) Botulinum toxin a has antinociceptive effects in treating interstitial cystitis. Urology 64(5):871–875; discussion 875

Tirumuru S, Al-Kurdi D, Latthe P (2010) Intravesical botulinum toxin A injections in the treatment of painful bladder syndrome/interstitial cystitis: a systematic review. Int Urogynecol J 21:1285–1300

Zermann D, Ishigooka M, Schubert J, Schmidt RA (2000) Perisphincteric injection of botulinum toxin type A. A treatment option for patients with chronic prostatic pain? Eur Urol 38(4):393–399

Pediatric Botulinum Toxin Applications

6.1 Introduction

Children with detrusor overactivity, especially spina bifida and cerebral palsy kids, may also be good candidates for bladder botulinum toxin therapy. Effects on detrusor compliance, resolution of vesicoureteral reflux and/or hydronephrosis are some key questions raised when considering a child for bladder botulinum toxin injection (Schurch and Corcos 2005). This chapter focus on issues important for the use of botulinum toxin in pediatric population. We recommend the practitioner, especially those new to using botulinum toxin to read the (Chap. 3) neurogenic and (Chap. 4) idiopathic bladder chapters first. Consideration should be given to the appropriate dose of toxin in children, patient preparation and injection technique.

Children with neurogenic detrusor overactivity (NDO), especially those with myelodysplasia, are potential candidates for bladder BoNT therapy. There are several studies in pediatric patients demonstrating the safety and efficacy of BoNT. However, pediatric detrusor overactivity was not included in international registry trials.

Two especially important issues that always come up in discussion of pediatric indications are the risk of vesicoureteral reflux with BoNT injection and if decreased detrusor compliance in myelodysplastic patients is a contraindication. One can ask two questions. First, will BoNT cause vesicoureteral reflux or can it improve reflux? Second, can BoNT improve a neurogenic bladder that has abnormal compliance or does it depend upon whether the poor compliance is due to increased neurogenic tone or increased fibrosis? Our experience and some recent studies show that not only does BoNT does not cause vesicoureteral reflux but may improve or resolve the ureteral reflux (Smith and Chancellor 2004) (Fig. 6.1). There is also data to suggest that BoNT can improve even the poorly compliant bladder and may be an effective alternative option to bladder augmentation.

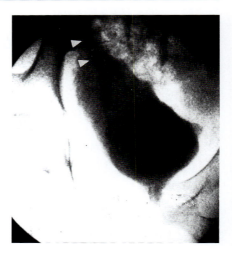

Fig. 6.1 Voiding cystourethrogram in a 12-year-old spina bifida boy demonstrating right vesicoureteral reflux. Bladder deviated to right side most likely from the constipation that the child also complains of and wishes to stop his antimuscarinic drugs

Table 6.1 Common pediatric neurological conditions associated with neurogenic bladder dysfunction
- Myelomeningocele
- Spina bifida
- Tethered cord syndrome and short filum terminale
- Cerebral palsy

6.2 Indications

Some of the most common neurological conditions that will be encountered for children who may be candidates for botulinum toxin injection include spina bifida, myelomeningocele, tethering of the cord, or sacral anomalies and cerebral palsy. In most cases, the defect will be apparent at birth (Table 6.1). Only occasionally will older children with tethering of the cord come to the attention of the clinician with spina bifida occulta with such manifestations as skin discoloration and abnormal hair growth or a sacral dimple of the lower spine area.

Special Emphasis: It should be remembered that the majority of data on botulinum toxin injection for neurogenic detrusor overactivity are from the two groups of neurogenic detrusor overactivity patients, spinal cord injury and multiple sclerosis, included in the registry trials for regulatory approval. There is no regulatory trial for pediatric indication at this time.

6.2.1 When to Consider Botulinum Toxin Injection

Failure with conservative approach with antimuscarinic drugs, revealed by recurrent leakage, recurrent urinary tract infection, or persistent or worsening of hydronephrosis, suggests that one considers alternative treatment. Up to now, only surgery in the form of various types of bladder augmentation was proposed to preserve renal function, and to promote low storage bladder pressure and continence. There is increasing evidence that botulinum toxin may be an effective treatment for children with detrusor overactivity.

6.2.2 Nonneurogenic Indications in Children

Beside the classic neurogenic detrusor overactivity, there are studies that report efficacy with bladder injection for children with idiopathic detrusor overactivity and sphincter injection for children with voiding dysfunction. We will review the results in Sect. 6.5 for the neon-neurogenic indications in children.

6.3 What Is the Work-Up?

6.3.1 History and Physical Examination

One should do a complete history including symptoms related to the birth history, neurologic injury or disease. Past medical history including medical and surgical history is required and response to any medications, especially if they have had BoNT in the past. Urogenital issues including bladder diary and fecal continence status should be addressed. Neurogenic functional status, ambulation status and hand dexterity are of particular importance. Catheter usage and the ability to do catheterization is a high priority before considering BoNT. Home and social setting play a role in developing a realistic plan including school arrangement and family's interest. The risk for latex allergy should be considered.

6.3.2 Urodynamic Evaluation

Ultrasound and urodynamics in conjunction with evaluation of leakage episodes and recurrent infections are key elements for adequate management. In most cases, basic treatment is composed of intermittent catheterization and anticholinergic agents (Joseph et al. 1989; Edelstein et al. 1995).

Urodynamic testing plays a pivotal role in evaluating patients with neurogenic bladder. This is a valuable tool to establish baseline bladder pressures and behavior that can be used for the diagnosis, prognosis, and management of their disease (Bauer et al. 1984). Annual urodynamic studies are often recommended to assess disease process changes, especially in those with febrile infection, high bladder pressures, poor bladder compliance, or hydronephrosis or reflux. Urodynamic parameters recorded include: bladder sensation, filling pressure, capacity, compliance, uninhibited detrusor contractions, and residual volume.

Urodynamic evaluation is essential makes pattern recognition possible and helps to establish a management plan for each patient. In general the combination of detrusor overactivity and sphincter spasticity is potentially dangerous because of high intravesical pressures, putting the upper tract at risk; whereas' an inactive detrusor or a paralyzed sphincter, providing a low pressure reservoir, is relatively safe.

Renal hydronephrosis and vesicoureteral reflux should be ruled out using ultrasound and voiding cystogram. If any imaging reveals abnormalities or if the bladder does not empty properly, early intermittent catheterization should be instituted. Recurrent infections could also be an indication of the early need for intermittent catheterization.

6.4 How to Do It

Please see neurogenic detrusor overactivity (Chap. 3) on patient preparation, reconstitution; injection technique and follow-up as they are similar in adult and children with neurogenic detrusor overactivity. Special attention and precaution should be given to the high incidence of Latex allergy in spina bifida children although small cystoscopic equipment may be required.

6.4.1 Cystoscope

Both rigid pediatric and flexible cystoscopic techniques work well in our hands and those of most experts without an apparent difference in clinical outcomes. Clinician's preference and institutional practice usually decide what technique is used. In children sedation is often necessary so use of a rigid cystoscope with small caliber endoscopic needle may be more appropriate.

Flexible Scope: We prefer (MBC) prefers using the flexible scope as the preferred injection technique for both males and females children. The flexible scope accommodates a 27 Fr flexible Olympus® injection needle (disposable) which must be passed through a reusable sheath. Office procedures with only local anesthesia are adequate for some of our patients. Although the same technique can be applied with sedation in a hospital setting. (Fig. 6.2).

The bladder volume is typically kept at 150–200 ml in adult but is likely to be less in children. We prefer to have the bladder moderately full to best visualize the entire inner surface. Blood vessels are avoided during injection. The first observable change is in urgency, frequency, and incontinence after 4–7 days, and all variables improve significantly after 4 weeks.

6.4.2 Botulinum Toxin Reconstitution

Each vial of 100 U onabotulinumtoxinA (Botox®, Allergan Inc., Irvine, CA) is usually reconstituted to 10 ml with injectable preservative-free saline, making the concentration

Fig. 6.2 Cystogram illustrating severe bladder trabeculation, a common finding in myelodysplastic children with neurogenic detrusor overactivity. The bladder capacity is decreased and the detrusor wall thickened with trabeculation. A flexible cystoscope can be seen in the bladder in preparation for botulinum toxin injection

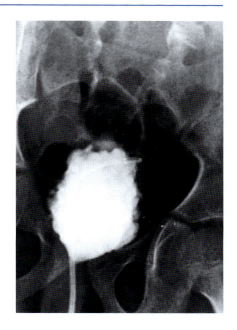

equivalent to 10 U/ml. OnabotulinumtoxinA is kept in the refrigerator according to instruction and we usually do not reconstitute the onabotulinumtoxinA until we know that infection has been ruled out or an appropriate antibiotic started to avoid wastage.

Each vial of abobotulinumtoxinA (Dysport®; Ipsen Ltd., Berkshire, UK) contains either 300 U (i.e., for glabellar lines) or 500 U (i.e., for cervical dystonia). Studies have documented dilutions with preservative-free saline to a concentration of 25–100 U/ml.

Each vial of rimabotulinumtoxinB (Myobloc and Neurobloc®, US WorldMeds, Louisville, KY) contains 5,000 U/ml and, as opposed to onabotulinumtoxinA (i.e., vacuum-dried) and abobotulinumtoxinA (i.e., freeze-dried) preparations, is already reconstituted. Although few studies have used rimabotulinumtoxinB to treat bladder overactivity, most have diluted to a concentration of 250 U/ml.

6.4.3 Dose

For pediatric patients, we generally start with no more than 100 U dose of onabotulinumtoxinA and less in smaller children and those with multiple medical problems. Some series have described doses up to 12 U/kg, similar to doses given in other neuropediatric populations (Schulte-Baukloh et al. 2002a). Typical doses in adult patients treated with abobutulinumtoxinA range between 500 and 1,000 U, and for rimabotulinumtoxinB range between 2,500 and 15,000 U (i.e., 5,000 U most common).

The potency units of all commercially available BoNTs are specific to that particular preparation and assay method utilized. They are not interchangeable with other preparations of BoNT products. Units of biological activity of one toxin preparation cannot be compared or converted into units of any other botulinum toxin products.

6.4.4 Depth, Location, and Amount of Injection

We usually inject 1 ml/site (10 U onabotulinumtoxinA/ml) so, for example, if we are using 100 U there will be approximately ten injection sites (Smith and Chancellor 2005). If we were to use 200 U of onabotulinumtoxinA for a 16 year-old spina bifida boy with body mass index of 30, we would take two bottles of 100 U of onabotulinumtoxinA and dissolve each bottle in 10 ml of preservative-free saline and inject into 20 sites of 1 ml each.

6.4.5 Injection Technique

How deep should BoNT be injected into the bladder? Recent evidence in human cadaveric bladder tissues demonstrates that the botulinum toxin-A receptor co-localizes with parasympathetic nerves within the suburothelium and detrusor muscle. Thus, both detrusor and urothelial injection are appropriate. Kuo demonstrated significant increases in functional bladder capacity, and significant reductions in urge episodes without an increase in post-void residual in patients with idiopathic overactive bladder undergoing bladder trigone sub-urothelial injections compared to patients injected intramuscularly outside of the trigone (Kuo 2007).

We were the first to suggest that bladder BoNT injection consider urothelial delivery to potentially target the suburothelial sensory pathway rather than paralysis of the detrusor in the treatment of the overactive bladder (Smith and Chancellor 2004). Injection into the suburothelium might avoid the potential loss of BoNT through detrusor injections and allow for lower doses and more refined injection paradigms to be employed. However, in many neurogenic detrusor overactivity patients who are already catheterizing and where complete paralysis is the treatment objective, perhaps deeper detrusor injections should be the approach used. Unfortunately, especially in idiopathic detrusor overactivity bladders and particularly in children with a thin bladder wall, it might be difficult to differentiate suburothelium from detrusor muscle.

6.4.5.1 Trigone Injection

A successful outcome was reported with BoNT injection into only the trigone and bladder base (Smith and Chancellor 2005). The rationale for trigone injection is that this portion of the urinary bladder contains a prominent parasympathetic plexus of BoNT receptor-positive nerves. This also does not take into account a possible therapeutic effect of BoNT on the abundant sensory nerves within the trigone. Although vesicoureteral reflux might be a potential complication after BoNT with trigonal injection, there is no clinical evidence of it so far (Smith et al. 2005; Chancellor 2010). In the present authors' personal experience over the past 10 years, submucosal trigone and bladder base injections of BoNT are associated with a low incidence of urinary retention and a similar efficacy to intradetrusor injection.

It should be emphasized that no standardized injection technique exists for BoNT injection in lower urinary tract tissues. Different bladder injection paradigms have been described (i.e., trigone vs. trigone-sparing) although none has been proven to be superior to the other.

6.4.6 Post-procedure and Follow-up

We instruct our patient's that they may notice some pain and blood-tinged urine, as well as possible difficulty urinating following treatment. These symptoms should resolve within 24 h and they should call and contact us immediately if they have any questions or concerns. We discuss the appropriate antibiotic coverage and risk of infection in these patients who often have more bladder infections. For those who are not already on intermittent catheterization, we formulate a plan if urinary retention occurs.

Results of botulinum toxin injection are not instantaneous. It may take several days to notice a gradual improvement in overactive bladder symptoms. Similarly, it generally takes several days for a patient to notice impaired voiding and we would instruct that patient to start self-catheterization if clinically necessary (Fig. 6.3).

6.5 What Are the Results?

There are only a few studies that have evaluated the efficacy of botulinum toxin injection in a pediatric neurogenic population with neurogenic detrusor overactivity. Schulte-Baukloh et al. (2002a, 2003) injected 20 myelodysplastic children with neurogenic detrusor overactivity with 12 U/kg (maximum 300 U onabotulinumtoxinA). Urodynamic follow-up at 2–4 weeks after treatment revealed 35% increases in maximal bladder capacity and significant decreases in maximal detrusor pressure (41% decline). However, while significant augmentation of maximum bladder capacity was demonstrated up to 6 months after treatment, no significant difference in maximum detrusor pressure was seen at 3–6 month follow-up (Case Study 6.1 and Fig. 6.4).

Schulte-Baukloh and associates (2002b) reported 17 children (average age 10.8 years) who had detrusor hyperreflexia and were using clean intermittent catheterization four or five times a day. Urodynamic studies were followed by injection of 85–300 U of onabotulinumtoxinA toxin into 30–40 sites in the detrusor muscle. Urodynamic follow-up was done 2–4 weeks after injection.

Fig. 6.3 Cystogram 3 months after BoNT in same child as in Fig. 6.2 demonstrating increased bladder capacity and decreased trabeculation

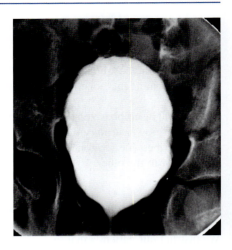

Case Study 6.1: A 17-year-old spina bifida girl with persistent urinary incontinence

Chief Complaint: Urinary incontinence despite large doses of antimuscarinics that causes dry mouth and constipation.

A 17-year-old spina bifida girl who wets two large diapers a day despite 30 mg of oxybutynin/day and intermittent self-catheterization approximately every 2–3 h. Patient is highly bothered by dry mouth and constipation caused by her antimuscarinic drugs. Parents and child are worried about smell and control of leakage as she is planning to attend college. They are leaning toward augmentation cystoplasty but were hoping to avoid major surgery.

Treatment: 200 U onabotulinumtoxinA injection into 20 spots in the bladder, including trigone.

Urodynamics before and after treatment is illustrated in Fig. 6.4. Cystometrogram before (top panel) and 6 months (*bottom panel*) after 200 U onabotulinumtoxinA injection. At baseline (*top panel*) the Pves increased to a volume of 240 ml where she leaked at a pressure of 48 cmH$_2$O.

Outcome: 6 months after onabotulinumtoxinA the bladder compliance significantly improved with decreased filling pressure to a volume of 500 ml of only 15 cmH$_2$O. The patient reported minimal leakage needing only one small pad per day; she takes 10 mg oxybutynin/day and can self-catheterize at a frequency of every 4–6 h. Nine months after the botulinum toxin injection, the girl and her mom noticed her capacity had decreased, and she had a few more episodes of incontinence and she requested retreatment.

6.5 What Are the Results?

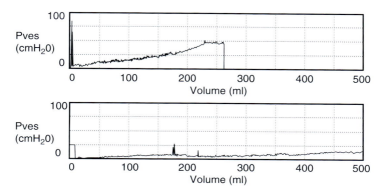

Fig. 6.4 Cystometrogram before (*top panel*) and 6 months (*bottom panel*) after 200 U onabotulinumtoxinA injection in case study. Pves: intravesical pressure (cm H_2O)

The mean reflex volume increased by 112%, from 95 to 201 mL ($P<0.005$). The maximal bladder capacity increased by 57%, from 138 to 215 mL ($P<0.005$). The maximal detrusor pressure decreased by 33%, from 59 to 40 cmH$_2$O ($P<0.005$). Detrusor compliance increased by 122%, from 20 to 45 mL/cmH$_2$O ($P<0.01$).

Another series with longer follow-up in 15 patients (mean age 5.8 years) demonstrated a 118% increase of maximal bladder capacity and a 46% decline of maximal detrusor pressure with onabotulinumtoxinA injection (Riccabona et al. 2004). The clinical effects lasted a mean of 10.5 months and were maintained with after repeated injections. No adverse events related to the toxin or to the injection procedure were reported in these two studies.

Corcos and associates (2004) reported on repeated injection in a population of 20 myelodysplastic children (average age 13 years); they showed after the first injection that maximal bladder capacity increased from 198 to 285 mL, maximum detrusor pressure decreased from 45 to 30 cmH$_2$O, and compliance rose from 5 to 13 mL/cmH$_2$O. After the second and subsequent treatments (up to four) a similar range of improvement was observed for these three parameters.

Neel and colleagues (2007) investigated if botulinum toxin may be better used alone or in conjunction with oxybutynin chloride in the management of 23 refractory neuropathic bladder children (average age 5.6 years). Patients were randomly assigned into two groups. Group 1 (12 patients) continued to receive oxybutynin while in group 2 (11 patients), anticholinergics were discontinued. Clinical and urodynamic evaluations were performed before injection, and at 1- and 6-month intervals. Patients were then followed every 6 months with urodynamic study.

Maximum bladder capacity increased from 96 to 163 mL at 1 month and to 142 mL at 6 months. Maximal detrusor pressure decreased from 76 to 50 and 51 cmH$_2$O at 1 and 6 months, respectively. Nine of the 16 incontinent patients (56%) showed complete continence after treatment, while four (25%) reported mild to moderate improvement and three (19%) showed no improvement. None of the patients had side effects related to the procedure or the material used. Neel et al. (2007) concluded that there is beneficial use of botulinum-A toxin for the treatment of refractory neuropathic bladder and have not yet found any augmentative effect of oxybutynin chloride in this study group. Accordingly, we can use such a modality as sole treatment for noncompliant neuropathic bladder.

6.5.1 Idiopathic Detrusor Overactivity Clinical Studies

Botulinum toxin treatment of children with idiopathic detrusor overactivity has been reported (Verleyen et al. 2004). Eleven children, mean age 10 years, with detrusor overactivity and daytime incontinence who had failed medical therapy were injected with either 125 or 250 U of onabotulinumtoxinA. The authors reported an increase in functional bladder capacity, with a reduction in idiopathic detrusor overactivity contractions and urgency symptoms. However, one girl needed to perform self-catheterizations for 2 weeks after injection.

Hoebeke et al. (2006) determined the effect of detrusor injection of botulinum-A toxin in a cohort of children (10 boys and 11 girls) with therapy resistant non-neurogenic detrusor overactivity. All patients showed decreased bladder capacity for age, urge and urge incontinence. Main treatment duration before inclusion was 45 months. A dose of 100 U onabotulinumtoxinA was injected in the detrusor.

Eight girls and seven boys with a minimum follow-up of 6 months represent the study group for long-term evaluation. In this study group after one injection, nine patients showed full response (no more urge and dry during the day) with a mean increase in bladder capacity from 167 to 271 ml. Three patients showed a partial response (50% decrease in urge and incontinence) and three remained unchanged. Eight of the nine full responders were still cured after 12 months, while one of the initially successfully treated patients had relapse after 8 months. The three partial responders and the patient with relapse underwent a second injection with a full response in the former full responder and in one partial responder.

Side effects reported include one girl with 10 days of temporary urinary retention and clinical signs of vesicoureteral reflux with flank pain during voiding in one boy that disappeared spontaneously after 2 weeks. No further examinations were done since the boy refused. Two girls experienced one episode each of symptomatic lower urinary tract infection.

6.5.2 Voiding Dysfunction Clinical Studies

Radojicic et al. (2006) assessed BoNT in children with voiding dysfunction via transperineal pelvic floor/external sphincter injection combined with behavioral and biofeedback reeducation in children with voiding dysfunction who had been resistant to previously applied therapies. Eight boys and 12 girls between 7 and 12 years old (mean age 9) with recurrent urinary tract infection, an interrupted or fractional voiding pattern and high post-void residual urine in whom behavioral, shortern biofeedback and alpha-blocker therapies had failed were included in the study. They were treated with 50–100 U onabotulinumtoxinA injected transperineally into the pelvic floor and/or external sphincter.

In boys, the sphincter was localized endoscopically before injection (endoscopically assisted transperineal approach). Behavioral and biofeedback reeducation started 15 days after injection. Follow-up was between 9 and 14 months. All patients were without urinary tract infection and fever, while five were still on chemoprophylaxis. Six months after treatment residual urine decreased in 17 of 20 patients. Nine patients reestablished a normal voiding curve and eight showed improvement. Three did not manifest any significant improvement. In one girl transitory incontinence resolved spontaneously within 48 h. There were no other complications.

The authors reported that although the effect of botulinum toxin injection is transitory, its muscle relaxation may break the circle of detrusor-sphincter dyssynergia, and the period when it is sustained can be used for retraining the patient in normal voiding.

Mokhless et al. (2006) evaluated onabotulinumtoxinA injection into the urethral sphincter in children with nonneurogenic neurogenic bladder to decrease urethral resistance and improve voiding. In these patients, alpha-blocker medications had failed and injection was an alternative to unavailable biofeedback.

Prospective treatment was performed in ten children 6–17 years old (mean age 8) with nonneurogenic neurogenic bladder using onabotulinumtoxinA. Preoperatively all children were evaluated by ultrasound, voiding cystourethrography, excretory urography, magnetic resonance imaging and urodynamic studies, including pressure flow, electromyography and uroflowmetry. One patient had unilateral and four had bilateral hydronephrosis. Using a rigid pediatric endoscope and a 4 Fr injection needle 50–100 U onabotulinumtoxinA were injected into the external sphincter at the 3, 6 and 9 o'clock positions. Follow-up was 6–15 months. Repeat injections every month were given according to the response with a maximum of three injections.

Immediately after botulinum toxin injection, all except one patient were able to void without catheterization. No acute complications occurred. Four patients with bilateral hydronephrosis and the patient with the refluxing unit showed regression. Postoperatively post-void residual urine decreased by 89%, detrusor leak point pressure decreased significantly from a mean 66 to 37 cmH$_2$O and uroflowmetry showed an increase in maximum urine flow from 2 to 18 mL/s after injection. Three injections were needed in one patient to attain the desired response. Urethral sphincter botulinum-A toxin injection could be considered a reliable treatment modality in children with nonneurogenic neurogenic bladder after the failure of conservative therapy.

6.5.3 Repeat Injection

To assess the long-term success of treatment with repeated onabotulinumtoxinA injections into the detrusor muscle for neurogenic detrusor overactivity in children, Schulte-Baukloh et al. (2005) reviewed the charts of ten children (average age at first injection 11.2 years) with neurogenic detrusor overactivity who had received at least three onabotulinumtoxinA detrusor injections; four had received five or more injections. The total dose of onabotulinumtoxinA was 85–300 U. Urodynamics were assessed 6 months after each injection and results after the first injection were compared with the results after the third and fifth injections (in the children who had five or more injections).

The relative changes – each in comparison with the value before injection therapy – after the first versus the fifth injection were as follows: the reflex volume increased by 81% versus 88%, maximal detrusor pressure decreased by 7% versus 39%, maximal cystometric bladder capacity increased by 88% versus 72%, and bladder compliance showed no change at the 6-month follow-up visit after the first injection and an increase of 109% after the fifth injection. The results after the third injection were generally similar to those after the fifth injection. No major side effects occurred.

Although this is a small case series, the efficacy was promising and noticeable changes in urodynamic parameters after repeated BoNT detrusor injections in children with neurogenic bladder were observed. There was no evidence of drug tolerance or antibody formation.

6.6 Conclusions

It has been over a decade since we started using botulinum toxin in selected patients and in registered clinical trials. We have seen remarkable improvement in bladder function when high doses of anticholinergics simply are not enough or the side effect versus benefit ratio is not sufficient. We have seen resolution of vesicoureteral reflux and improvement of decreased detrusor compliance. Most importantly, we have seen neurologically impaired children spared from more invasive reconstructive surgery. Careful, watchful waiting may be considered if botulinum toxin maintains normal renal function, prevents febrile urinary tract infection and protects the upper urinary tract while giving the child and his/her family adequate control and improved quality of life.

References

Bauer SB, Hallett M, Khoshbin S et al (1984) Predictive value of urodynamic evaluation in newborns with myelodysplasia. JAMA 252:650–652

Chancellor MB (2010) Ten years single surgeon experience with botulinum toxin in the urinary tract; clinical observations and research discovery. Int Urol Nephrol 42:383–391

Corcos J, Al-Taweed W, Robichaud C (2004) Botulinum toxin as an alternative treatment to bladder augmentation in children with neurogenic bladder due to myelomeningocele [abstract]. J Urol 171:181

Edelstein RA, Bauer SB, Kelly MD et al (1995) The long-term urological response of neonates with myelodysplasia treated proactively with intermittent catheterization and anticholinergic therapy. J Urol 154:1500–1504

Hoebeke P, De Caestecker K, Vande Walle J, Dehoorne J, Raes A, Verleyen P, Van Laecke E (2006) The effect of botulinum-A toxin in incontinent children with therapy resistant overactive detrusor. J Urol 176:328–330; discussion 330–331

Joseph DB, Bauer SB, Colodny AH et al (1989) Clean, intermittent catheterization of infants with neurogenic bladder. Pediatrics 84:78–82

Kuo HC (2007) Comparison of effectiveness of detrusor, suburothelial and bladder base injections of botulinum toxin a for idiopathic detrusor overactivity. J Urol 178:1359–1363

Mokhless I, Gaafar S, Fouda K, Shafik M, Assem A (2006) Botulinum A toxin urethral sphincter injection in children with nonneurogenic neurogenic bladder. J Urol 176:1767–1770; discussion 1770

Neel KF, Soliman S, Salem M, Seida M, Al-Hazmi H, Khatab A (2007) Botulinum-A toxin: solo treatment for neuropathic noncompliant bladder. J Urol 178:2593–2597; discussion 2597–2598

Radojicic ZI, Perovic SV, Milic NM (2006) Is it reasonable to treat refractory voiding dysfunction in children with botulinum-A toxin? J Urol 176:332–336; discussion 336

Riccabona M, Koen M, Schindler M et al (2004) Botulinum-A toxin injection into the detrusor: a safe alternative in the treatment of children with myelomeningocele with detrusor hyperreflexia. J Urol 171:845–848

Schulte-Baukloh H, Knispel HH, Michael T (2002a) Botulinum-A toxin in the treatment of neurogenic bladder in children. Pediatrics 110:420–421

Schulte-Baukloh H, Michael T et al (2002b) Efficacy of botulinum-a toxin in children with detrusor hyperreflexia due to myelomeningocele: preliminary results. Urology 59:325–327; discussion 327–328

Schulte-Baukloh H, Michael T, Sturzebecher B, Knispel HH (2003) Botulinum-a toxin detrusor injection as a novel approach in the treatment of bladder spasticity in children with neurogenic bladder. Eur Urol 44:139–143

Schulte-Baukloh H, Knispel HH, Stolze T, Weiss C, Michael T, Miller K (2005) Repeated botulinum-A toxin injections in treatment of children with neurogenic detrusor overactivity. Urology 66:865–870

Schurch B, Corcos J (2005) Botulinum toxin injections for paediatric incontinence. Curr Opin Urol 15:264–267

Smith CP, Chancellor MB (2004) Emerging role of botulinum toxin in the management of voiding dysfunction. J Urol 171:2128–2137

Smith CP, Chancellor MB (2005) Simplified bladder botulinum-toxin delivery technique using flexible cystoscope and 10 sites of injection. J Endourol 19:880–882

Smith CP, Nishiguchi J et al (2005) Single-institution experience in 110 patients with botulinum toxin A injection into bladder or urethra. Urology 65:37–41

Verleyen P, Hoebeke P, Raes P et al (2004) The use of botulinum toxin A in children with a nonneurogenic overactive bladder: a pilot study. BJU Int 93(suppl):69–72

Part III
Prostate and Pelvic Floor

Botulinum Toxin Injection for Prostate Disorders

7.1 Introduction

Benign prostatic hyperplasia (BPH) with its related symptoms is a common condition that affects nearly half of men over age 50 and 90% of men over the age of 80 (McVary 2006). Lower urinary tract symptoms caused by BPH which include nocturia, frequency, urgency, hesitancy, intermittency, and incomplete emptying can be very bothersome, affect an individual's lifestyle significantly, and are costly (Wei et al. 2005). The condition is associated with a reduced quality of life and sleep disturbance. BPH may lead to urinary retention, bladder stones, renal insufficiency, and urinary tract infections. The anatomical location of the human prostate and the urethra lend itself to the development of lower urinary tract symptoms including both obstructive and irritative symptoms. The initial evaluation of BPH includes administration of a validated symptom index that evaluates the presence and severity of the main components of lower urinary tract symptoms. The importance of symptoms in the pathophysiology of BPH is underscored by the fact that symptom measurements comprised 78% of all endpoints from the recent Medical Treatment of Prostate Symptoms trial, compared to 22% of endpoints for objective measures such as urinary retention and urinary tract infection (Gormley et al. 2002). BPH, in a large part, is a neural phenomenon given that sensory symptoms such as frequency, urgency, and nocturia are key factors that push patients to seek treatment.

Expert Opinion: The Ideal Candidates for BoNT Prostate Injection
Yao-Chi Chuang, M.D.
  Associate Professor and Director of Urology
  Chang Gung Memorial Hospital Kaohsiung, Taiwan
  Lower urinary tract symptoms suggestive of benign prostatic hyperplasia (BPH) are frequently encountered in aging men. In addition to medical treatment and surgical ablation of obstructive prostate, there has been much interest in the

development of minimally invasive treatments for BPH. Among them, intraprostatic injection therapy for BPH has been explored to reduce prostate volume since the early 1900s.

BoNT acting at the nerve terminals, blocking vesicle transport of neurotransmitters, including acetylcholine, noradrenalin, and sensory neuropeptides, can alter neural control of the prostate, and might relieve voiding symptoms independent of prostate size. Therefore, BoNT prostate injection represents an alternative option for the treatment of symptomatic BPH.

Many small series of studies on BoNT prostate injection therapy provide evidence that it may relieve symptoms for duration of approximately 9–12 months, and resume spontaneous voiding in some men with urinary retention. Nevertheless, there is less urodynamic evidence for its relief of obstruction and lack of large randomized double blind control studies to rule out the impact of placebo or prostate acupuncture effects. I have found that many men are willing to accept a once-a-year BoNT prostate injection if it reduces risks, avoids hospitalization, has a reliable efficacy, and does not cause retrograde ejaculation.

The ideal candidates for BoNT prostate injection in my experience have the following criteria:

- Lower urinary tract symptoms (International Prostate Symptom Score≥12) due to BPH for at least 6 months.
- Refractory to usage of an oral BPH drug (>4 week duration for alpha antagonists; >6 months duration for 5-alpha reductase inhibitors if prostate volume between 40 and 80 mL). If patients also have overactive bladder symptoms they should try an antimuscarinic agent for at least 1 month.
- Refractory BPH induced acute urinary retention and not willing or unfitted to receive surgical ablation of prostate.
- Patients with not excessively large prostate (<40 mL) and with decreased maximum flow rate <12 mL/s have done better.
- Rule out acute prostatitis or urinary tract infection.
- PSA level <4 mg/L and without clinical suspicious of prostate cancer.

Prostatic injections of BoNT can be carried out transperineally, transrectally, or transurethrally. I personally prefer the transperineal injection to minimize the risk of infection and I can do it without anesthesia. Patients with large median lobe cannot be approached through the transperineal or transrectal injection. I typically use 200 U onabotulinumtoxinA to treat BPH. I mix the onabotulinumtoxinA with 4 mL sterile saline and under ultrasound guided I injection 2 mL (100 U each) onabotulinumtoxinA into each of the middle of the prostate on the right and left side.

Although clinical series demonstrates efficacy of minimum 6 months, more studies are necessary in order to identify the mechanisms by which BoNT affects the prostate, the ideal dose, and the duration of effect. Since the use of BoNT in the prostate is currently FDA off-label and, in support of evidence based medicine practices, caution should be applied until larger randomized clinical studies are completed.

7.2 Prostate BoNT Rationale and Mechanism of Action

While surgery remains the gold standard for relieving obstruction and symptoms, more recent attention has been focused on pharmacotherapy as an alternative approach. The American Urological Association recommends alpha-adrenergic receptor blockers as first-line pharmacologic therapy for male patients suffering from BPH. Alpha-adrenergic receptor blockers antagonize adrenergic receptors, blocking the effects of norepinephrine released from sympathetic nerve terminals. The end result is reduced smooth muscle tone. Numerous studies have documented a beneficial effect of alpha-adrenergic receptor blockers for improving lower urinary tract symptoms and urinary flow rates (Nickel et al. 2008). However, use of alpha-adrenergic receptor blockers can be associated with serious cardiovascular and sexual side effects that contribute to the fact that one-third of men discontinue drug use despite bothersome lower urinary tract symptoms (Verhamme et al. 2003). In addition, alpha-adrenergic receptor blockers directly target sympathetic pathways and ignore the contributory effect of parasympathetic innervation on prostate growth and lower urinary tract symptoms.

Increasing basic and clinical evidence suggests that neural pathways within the prostate modulate bladder storage function and may play a significant role in lower urinary tract symptoms. McVary and colleagues previously have demonstrated that surgical denervation of the rat prostate induces significant changes in the size of the rat ventral lobe (McVary et al. 1994). The effect of altered neural input on prostate growth was also evaluated in a population of partial and complete spinal cord injured men (Benaim et al. 1998). The study found no difference in prostate volume with increased age, a finding that contradicts observations from longitudinal studies in neurally intact males demonstrating that prostate size positively correlates with age. Given that no abnormalities in pituitary-gonadal axis were observed, it appears likely that loss of neural input resulting from spinal cord injury stunts prostate growth. These basic and clinical studies support further investigations evaluating the effect of targeted prostate denervation on male lower urinary tract symptoms associated with BPH.

In the search for more effective non-invasive therapies to treat BPH, the role of somatic and visceral neuromuscular activity in the manifestation of lower urinary tract symptoms has been studied (Lepor et al. 1987). BoNT injections have been reported to treat BPH (Chuang et al. 2006a; Maria et al. 2003) and other urologic disorders such as detrusor-sphincter dyssynergia, neurogenic detrusor over activity, chronic retention, chronic pelvic pain, and motor and sensory urinary urge incontinence (Smith 2009). BoNT's primary function is to inhibit the exocytosis of acetylcholine from the presynaptic nerve terminal. At greater doses, it can also block the release of other neurotransmitters including norepinephrine, substance P, calcitonin-gene related peptide, and glutamate (Chancellor et al. 2008).

When injected into rat prostates, BoNT has been shown to produce: (1) a generalized atrophy of the prostatic gland with no evidence of inflammatory infiltrate,

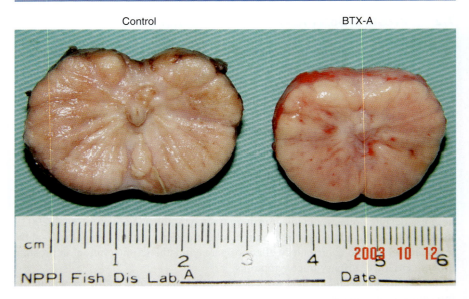

Fig. 7.1 Coronal section of canine prostate 1 month after saline or onabotulinumtoxinA injection. Note the significant decrease in size and induration after onabotulinumtoxinA injection compared to control prostates (Open access from Fig. 3 of Chuang et al. (2006c))

(2) an increase in apoptosis with DNA fragmentation and formation of apoptotic bodies on Tunnel stain and decrease in proliferation, (3) a reduction in the proliferation of epithelial cells, and (4) a reduction in alpha-1A adrenergic receptor but not androgen receptor expression (Figs. 7.1 and 7.2) (Chuang et al. 2006b; Doggweiler et al. 1998). Silva and associates found that BoNT induced prostate atrophy in rats could be prevented with daily injection of the adrenergic agonist phenylephrine but not from daily administration of the cholinergic agonist bethanechol (Silva et al. 2009b). Their investigations suggest that the predominant mechanism by which BoNT induces prostate atrophy and apoptosis in the rat is by inhibiting sympathetic neural transmission. Atrophy and apoptosis has also been observed in prostate tissues of dogs and humans following BoNT injection although the selective effect of BoNT on parasympathetic or parasympathetic pathways has not been evaluated in humans (Chuang et al. 2006c).

Based on the available literature and nonclinical studies, it is expected that intraprostatic BoNT will provide sustained symptomatic relief with minimal side effects. Besides its obvious efficacy in patients' refractory to alpha-1 adrenoceptor blocker therapy, BoNT injection has several potential advantages over oral agents. Focal prostate injection has been shown to be safe and obviates the systemic side effects observed with alpha-1 adrenoceptor blockers (i.e., orthostatic hypotension, sexual dysfunction). In addition, several studies demonstrate a durable response to BoNT treatment exceeding 12 months. This treatment may provide an important alternative option in the management of BPH without the need for daily pills and limiting systemic drug

7.3 Indications

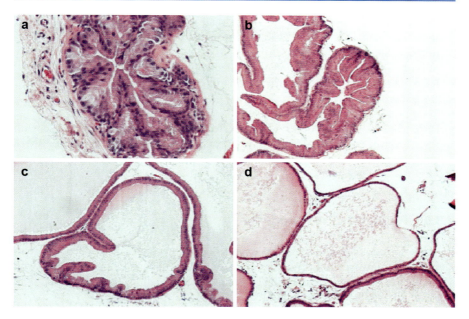

Fig. 7.2 Photomicrograph of prostate sections after saline (**a**), and 5 (**b**), 10 (**c**), and 20 U (**d**) of onabotulinumtoxinA treatment at 1 week. Significant glandular proliferation with papillary infolding in the lumen was seen in saline injected rat. Atrophy change in glandular component with flattening of lining epithelium was seen in onabotulinumtoxinA treated rat. Reduced from ×200 (Copyright obtained from Chuang et al. (2006b))

exposure. Furthermore, BoNT can be administered in the urologist's clinic without the use of general anesthesia, making it both convenient and practical.

7.3 Indications

7.3.1 BPH

General indication for BoNT prostate injection includes: history of lower urinary tract symptoms and signs suggestive of BPH and those previously failing treatment with oral BPH pharmacotherapy (alpha antagonists and/or 5-alpha reductase inhibitors). Clinical trials of BoNT BPH usually fit the following criteria and they are reasonable considerations for BoNT BPH candidates in our experience:
- Men aged 45 years or older.
- Lower urinary tract symptoms due to BPH for at least 6 months. For examples, most bothersome men will have International Prostate Symptom Score ≥14.
- Symptoms refractory to oral BPH drug (>4 week duration for alpha antagonists; >6 months duration for 5-alpha reductase inhibitors). Important that for men who are taking BPH oral drugs that they be on them for adequate duration to see if the drug works.

- Residual urine volume ≤200 mL. If residual volume is elevated we would perform urodynamic testing to evaluate detrusor contractility prior to BoNT injection consideration.
- Maximum flow rate ≤12 mL/s with voided volume ≥125 mL.
- Rule out acute prostatitis or urinary tract infection.
- Recent prostate biopsy.
- Total prostate volume less than 80 mL.
- PSA level <4 μg/L. Patients with elevated age adjusted PSA and those with PSA level of ≥4.0 μg/L should have prostate cancer ruled out prior to BoNT consideration.

7.3.2 Prostatitis/Prostatodynia

We have anecdotal positive clinical experience with prostate BoNT for the treatment of chronic abacterial prostatitis or prostatodynia. There are preclinical as well as small case series supporting BoNT use for these indications (Chuang et al. 2008; Maria et al. 1998; Zermann et al. 2000).

7.4 What Is the Work-up?

7.4.1 History and Physical Examination

A thorough history including symptoms related to BPH should be obtained. A specific medical and surgical history is required and response to any medications along with sexual history and voiding history. From over a decade of experience we have found men with symptomatic BPH but without excessively large glands (i.e., >80 g) are the best candidates.

We have found that men who had partial response to alpha blocker but stopped because not enough efficacy or not wanting to continue long-term alpha blocker; due to retrograde ejaculation and fatigue to be excellent prostate BoNT candidates. Contrary to some early publications on prostate BoNT, we have not found more than a 10–15% decrease in PSA or prostate volume. Urologists are trained and experienced with the work-up for BPH and lower urinary tract symptoms and we will not repeat the basic work-up here although all men should be screened for prostate cancer, when age appropriate.

Cystoscopy: Helpful to rule out median lobe enlargement which would be difficult to treat with BoNT prostate injection.

Urodynamic Evaluation: testing plays a helpful role in evaluating men with symptomatic BPH considering BoNT. This is a valuable tool to establish baseline bladder pressure and behavior that can be used for diagnosis, prognosis, and management. Pressure-flow study is the gold standard to diagnosis bladder outlet obstruction.

7.5 How to Do It

7.5.1 BPH

7.5.1.1 BoNT Reconstitution
Each vial of onabotulinumtoxinA contains 100 U of *Clostridium botulinum* toxin type A, 0.5 mg albumin (human) and 0.9 mg sodium chloride in a sterile, vacuum-dried form without a preservative. One unit corresponds to the calculated median lethal intraperitoneal dose in mice. We typically use 200 U of onabotulinumtoxinA for prostate indications diluted in a total volume of 4 mL of preservative-free saline.

7.5.1.2 Storage
OnabotulinumtoxinA should be stored in a secure area, accessible only to health care providers and administered only to patients entered into the clinic. The vacuum-dried vials of onabotulinumtoxinA should be stored in a refrigerator at 2–8°C until used. Reconstituted study medication must be stored in the vial or syringe in a refrigerator at 2–8°C and should be used within 24 h after reconstitution.

7.5.1.3 Preparation
We prepare the onabotulinumtoxinA only after the patient arrives in the clinic, has signed the informed consent, and has no contraindication to proceed with the injection. Two issues that have come up before are a positive pre-procedure urine analysis for bacteria and the patient did not stop anticoagulation therapy.

A total volume of 4 mL of onabotulinumtoxinA is prepared. When reconstituting onabotulinumtoxinA for each patient, preservative-free sterile saline should be injected gently into the onabotulinumtoxinA vial with a new syringe. The vacuum within the vial will draw in the saline. Do not use the vial if a vacuum is not observed. Once the saline has been drawn into the vial, the vial should be rotated gently to mix the contents. The reconstituted study medication should be clear, colorless, and free of particulate matter.

7.5.1.4 Prophylactic Antibiotics
Prior to injection, patients are prescribed an appropriate prophylactic antibiotic that should be started the day prior to treatment. The clinic should confirm that the patient has no known history of contraindications or resistance to the prescribed prophylactic antibiotic. The dosing regimen for the suggested antibiotics is as follows:
- Ciprofloxacin 500 mg twice daily for 4 days with the first dose taken 1 day prior to treatment.
- Depending on local antibiotic resistance pattern, a second generation cephalosporin, is becoming more widely used for prostate needle procedures. For these patients, the dosing regimen for suggested antibiotics is as follows: Cefuroxime or cefprozil 500 mg twice daily for 4 days with the first dose taken 1 day prior to

treatment. Other prophylactic antibiotics regimens can also be prescribed, at the physician's discretion, according to well-established local practices for transrectal or transperineal prostate biopsy. Aminoglycoside antibiotics should be avoided with BoNT procedures as they can impair neuromuscular function.

7.5.1.5 Pretreatment Enemas

Patients are to perform a rectal enema the morning of each treatment visit and the physician should be satisfied that the rectum is empty before proceeding with BoNT injection. A rectal suppository or laxative instead of a rectal enema is less desirable.

7.5.1.6 Equipment Preparation

The clinic should ensure that the rectal ultrasound probe and the needle guides or channels are clean and appropriately disinfected. Disposable guides and probe covers or sheaths are preferred, if available and suitable for the ultrasound probe.

7.5.1.7 Anesthesia

- Sterile single use local anesthetic gel (e.g., lidocaine gel) may be applied gently to the rectal wall overlying the prostate if the physician desires.
- Patients may receive sedation at the physician's discretion, if it is clinically indicated.
- In our experience, we have not found patients needing topical or injectable local anesthesia with prostate BoNT injection. Nor have our patients required sedation or oral analgesics before or after prostate BoNT injection.

7.5.1.8 Technique of Prostate BoNT Injection

Prostatic injections of BoNT can be carried out transperineally, transrectally, or transurethrally with preference often dictated by regional practice habits. Transperineal injection minimizes the risk of infection but ultrasound guided transrectal prostatic injection is the procedure that urologists are most familiar with in Europe and North America. The preparation and positioning of the patient is identical to that used for transrectal or transperineal ultrasound guided prostate biopsy (Fig. 7.3). Some urologists may prefer transurethral prostate injection using a familiar cystoscopy and injecting needle to approach the enlarged prostate glands (Fig. 7.4). This method may be more effective for managing trilobar prostate enlargement.

During treatment, onabotulinumtoxinA 200 U is reconstituted with normal saline to a volume of 4 mL or approximately 10% of total prostate volume or less and is injected at 2–4 locations. We use a 21–23 gauge 15 or 20 cm long needle under the guidance of transrectal ultrasound with the transverse and sagittal views to ensure proper placement of the needle as a bright spot in the center of each lateral lobe where 2 mL of BoNT is injected into each side or as described below in a numbered fashion for an injection into two separate spots in each lateral lobe. Diffusion of hyperechoic BoNT over the lateral lobe of the prostate can be easily seen with transrectal sonographic monitoring (Fig. 7.5).

Fig. 7.3 Transperineal intraprostatic BoNT injection under transrectal ultrasound guidance

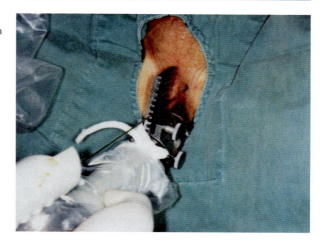

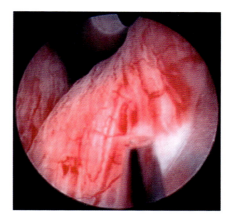

Fig. 7.4 Transurethral BoNT prostate injection: injection needle inserted into left lateral lobe

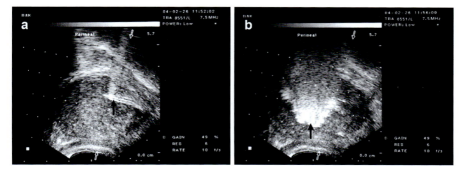

Fig. 7.5 (**a**) Confirmation of needle (*black arrow*) within the human prostate, longitudinal view. (**b**) Diffusion of hyperechoic onabotulinumtoxinA (*black arrow*) over the prostate immediate post injection (Open access from Fig. 2 of Chuang et al. (2006c))

7.5.1.9 Step-by-Step Four Quadrant Technique

1. The patient should be placed in the lateral decubitus position, facing away from the ultrasound monitor screen.
2. Sterile single use local anesthetic gel may be gently applied to the rectal wall digitally.
3. Ultrasound gel should be applied to the rectal probe or probe cover/sheath.
4. The rectal ultrasound probe should be gently inserted into the rectum.
5. Each prostate lobe will receive two injections (superior and inferior transition zone).
6. Using the ultrasound for guidance, advance the first needle to the cranial (superior) aspect of the first lateral lobe. The needle should be passed from posterior to anterior through the peripheral zone into the base of the prostate at the transition zone/central zone junction until it reaches the cranial aspect of the transition zone. The proper position should be approximately 1.0 cm from the bladder neck to avoid penetrating the bladder neck or bladder. If bladder neck or bladder penetration occurs, the needle should be repositioned. Care should also be taken to avoid the prostatic vessels, capsule, urethra, and sphincter.
7. A syringe should then be attached and the needle should be aspirated to ensure that there is no blood return (if there is blood return then the needle should be repositioned).
8. Following this, 1 mL of the BoNT should be injected into the superior (cranial aspect) of the transition zone.
9. The needle is then withdrawn to the inferior (caudal) aspect of the transition zone. The clinician should be assured that the needle tip is in the correct location within the inferior portion of the transition zone for administration.
10. The needle should again be aspirated to ensure that there is no blood return (if there is blood return then the needle should be repositioned).
11. A further 1 mL of the BoNT should be injected into the inferior (caudal) aspect of the transition zone.
12. Pause before removing the needle from the prostate lobe for at least 30 s following the caudal injection to avoid BoNT loss by leakage into the needle tract.
13. The identical procedure is performed on the contra lateral prostate lobe.
14. After the second lobe is injected and the needle removed, the rectal probe is also removed and the procedure is concluded.

7.5.1.10 Immediate Post-treatment Observation

Following injection, the patient should be observed until: he has voided and the clinic feels the patient's condition is sufficiently stable to be sent home. Prior to leaving the clinic, patients should be instructed to contact the health care team immediately if they experience any adverse events post-treatment. The patient should also be reminded to complete his course of prophylactic antibiotic medication.

7.5.2 Prostatitis/Prostatodynia

We have found that BoNT injections can be effective for reducing pain and incomplete emptying symptoms associated with non-bacterial prostatitis and prostatodynia. Patients typically describe pain in the penile or urethral area even though direct palpation reveals no abnormalities. However, digital rectal exam can often elicit the source of pain following compression of the prostate or external urethral sphincter/levator ani muscles. One technique we have found useful in localizing the source of pain and predicting response to BoNT injection is to first inject a local anesthetic into either the prostate or external urethral sphincter (i.e., depending on which site triggers pain with palpation). If both sites trigger pain, we will then sequentially inject local anesthesia on successive days.

A positive response, defined as a 50% or greater temporary reduction in pain symptoms, qualifies the patient to receive a subsequent injection with 100–200 U of onabotulinumtoxinA. Some patients with multifactorial pain symptoms receive injections in both their prostate and external urethral sphincter although we counsel them that they may suffer from transient stress urinary incontinence. We are careful with antibiotic coverage and men may stay on antibiotics for a longer-duration than following treatment for BPH.

7.6 What Are the Results?

Case Study 7.1: Man with symptomatic BPH but refuses surgical intervention
A 61-year-old man has slowly progressing lower urinary tract symptoms that are improved with oral tamsulosin 0.4 mg/day but he wants to stop the medicine due to adverse side effects. He is in excellent health, has a body mass index of 22 and runs mini-marathons. He eats an organic diet, and recently married for the second time to a younger woman. He notes that when he stops his alpha blocker, he has a stronger ejaculation and has more strength during exercise but his force of stream decreases significantly and his nocturia increases from 0–1 to 2–3 episodes per night. He does not want any surgery or irreversible procedures that may cause retrograde ejaculation. He did extensive research and decided that prostate BoNT would be an excellent option for him.

Pertinent Exam and Evaluation: Prostate is moderately enlarged without nodule and his PSA was 2.0 ng/dL. During Uroflow study, the patient voided 148 mL with a maximum flow rate of 9.0 mL/s and a post-void residual volume of 40 mL. Pressure-flow urodynamic study demonstrated high maximal detrusor voiding pressure and low flow rate (Fig. 7.6).

Treatment: The patient understood BoNT's off label use with unknown risks. He gave informed consent requesting procedure scheduling. The patient received

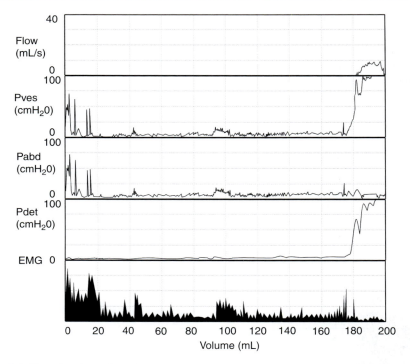

Fig. 7.6 Note the elevated maximum Pdet of nearly 100 cmH20 but with maximal flow rate of 8.8 mL/s during a voluntary detrusor contraction at approximately 180 mL. *Flow* uroflow rate mL/s, *Pves* Intravesical pressure, *Pabd* Intrabdominal pressure, *Pdet* Intradetrusor pressure: Pves – Pabd (cmH20), *EMG* electromyography

similar pre-procedure preparation for transrectal ultrasound guided BoNT injection as if he was having a prostate biopsy. Our current preparation and antibiotic coverage is listed in Sect. 4.1. BPH. No local anesthetic was used. Prostate volume was measured by transrectal ultrasound as 40 mL. Two-Hundred units of onabotulinumtoxinA was reconstituted in 4 mL of normal saline. A 23 G needle that we typically use for prostate local anesthetic injection was used.

The needle was inserted into each lobe and two injections (i.e., 100 U/injection) were performed.

Outcome: The patient did not report hematuria or hematospermia post injection. He noticed improvement in his voiding pattern after about 2 weeks and decided to stop his tamsulosin. He was pleased with his improved urination that he said "worked as good as the pill without taking a pill every day." Moreover, he noted "I am not as tired and my ejaculation is stronger."

7.6.1 BPH

The effect of onabotulinumtoxinA on lower urinary tract symptoms associated with BPH has been evaluated in several studies in men that have failed standard therapy with an alpha-adrenergic antagonist ± 5α-reductase inhibitor. The first off-label use of onabotulinumtoxinA to treat BPH in humans was reported by Maria et al. in 2003 (Maria et al. 2003). In a randomized, placebo-controlled study (i.e., evidence level 1b), 30 men with symptomatic BPH were randomized to receive either saline or 200 U of onabotulinumtoxinA. One hundred units of onabotulinumtoxinA in 2 mL of saline or saline alone were injected into each lobe of the prostate through the perineum via a 22 gauge spinal needle with transrectal ultrasound guidance.

Clinical improvement was evident within 1 month of treatment in the onabotulinumtoxinA group. By 2 months, 13 patients in the treatment group (87%) versus 3 patients in the control group (10%) reported subjective BPH symptom relief ($p=0.00001$). At 12 months, the International Prostate Symptom Score decreased by 62%, max urinary flow rate increased by 85%, post-void residual urine decreased by 85%, and prostate size (determined ultrasonographically) decreased by 61%. The PSA values were also reduced by 38%. This degree of improvement was remarkable considering the fact that most patients had severe baseline symptoms (average IPSS = 23) and the mean prostate size was large (i.e., 52 g) prior to injection. No urinary incontinence or systemic side effects were reported over the 19.6 month follow-up period.

Several case series have looked at specific BPH patient subpopulations to determine the effectiveness of onabotulinumtoxinA treatment. Kuo et al. treated ten patients who were either in frank urinary retention or carried a large post-void residual urine volume. These patients had already failed combination medical therapy (5α-reductase inhibitor and alpha-blocker) and were not surgical candidates due to comorbid medical conditions (Kuo 2005). Two hundred units of onabotulinumtoxinA was diluted in 10 mL of saline and was injected via a cystoscope into 10 sites in the prostate (4 sites on each lateral lobe, 2 sites at the median bar, 20 U per site). After onabotulinumtoxinA injection, seven of 10 patients (70%) could void spontaneously, while three required intermittent self-catheterization for 2 weeks. The therapeutic effects were experienced as early as 1 week after injection. By 3 and 6 months, significant improvements in maximal flow rate, residual urine volume, and prostate volumes were noted (53%, 85%, and 24%, respectively). Eight of ten patients continued to use combination medical therapy after onabotulinumtoxinA injection to maintain good symptomatic relief.

Chuang et al. stratified patients who had failed medical treatment based on the prostate size: those with <30 g were treated with 100 U onabotulinumtoxinA while those with >30 g were treated with 200 U (perineal injection) (Chuang et al. 2005; Chuang et al. 2006a). At 12 months, the percent improvements in International Prostate Symptom Score, maximum flow rate, and post-void residual urine volume were very similar to those of Maria et al., except that the percent shrinkage of prostate size was substantially smaller (13–19% versus 61%) (Table 7.1). In 12 of

Table 7.1 Results at 1, 3, 6, and 12 months in 20 men treated with 200 U onabotulinumtoxinA (Adapted from Chuang et al. (2006a))

Results at 1, 3, 6 and 12 Month in 20 Men Treated with 200 U BoNT-A

	Baseline (N=20)	1 M (N=20)	3M (N=17)	6M (N=15)	12M (N=11)
IPSS	19.3 ± 1.2	9.5 ± 2.0*	8.3 ± 2.0*	5.2 ± 1.1*	8.3 ± 1.9*
QOL	4.1 ± 0.2	2.0 ± 0.3*	2.2 ± 0.4*	1.8 ± 0.2*	2.4 ± 0.6*
Qmax	7.0 ± 1.1	10.3 ± 1.1*	9.8 ± 1.1*	11.9 ± 0.9*	11.1 ± 0.9*
RU	161.7 ± 48.1	45.2 ± 8.2*	37.6 ± 5.9*	45.5 ± 0.9*	93.6 ± 36.1
Prostate	54.3 ± 4.7	46.3 ± 3.7*	45.0 ± 4.2*	45.3 ± 4.1*	47.2 ± 4.0*

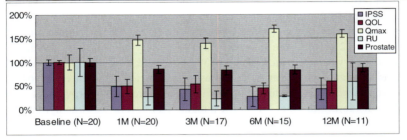

41 men (29%) there was no change in prostate volume, yet 7 of these 12 men (58%) still had a >30% improvement in International Prostate Symptom Score, maximum flow rate, and post-void residual urine volume, suggesting that onabotulinumtoxinA may relieve BPH symptoms by its effect on sensory nerve pathways rather than reducing the prostate size alone.

Our site (CPS) was one of seven centers involved in a 12-week Phase II trial of 100 and 300 U of onabotulinumtoxinA for the management of BPH (McVary et al. 2010). A total of 134 men were enrolled and treated (68 at dose 100 U and 66 at dose 300 U). One hundred twenty five men provided complete primary outcome data (63 at dose 100 U and 62 at dose 300 U). A positive effect of onabotulinumtoxinA was characterized as a ≥30% change from baseline in AUA Symptom Score (AUASS) and/or maximum flow rate. Both arms passed the efficacy criteria: 73% passed at the 100 U dose and 81% passed at the 300 U dose. Interestingly, no significant changes in total prostate volume or transition zone volume in the combined data of 100 U and 300 U (i.e., total prostate volume increased slightly from 49.7 g to 50.1 g and transition zone volume increased slightly from 24 g to 24.4 g) were observed. In addition, PSA values did not change significantly as a result of onabotulinumtoxinA treatment (i.e., increased non-significantly from 2.4 to 2.7 at 12 weeks follow-up).

Our results are consistent with other clinical studies of onabotulinumtoxinA in BPH although the 3-month improvements in AUASS (38% for 100 U dose; 46% for 300 U dose) and maximum flow rate (25% and 27%, respectively) demonstrated in our study were smaller than those described in prior studies (i.e., AUASS decrease

Table 7.2 Studies of BoNT for BPH

Investigator	Study type, N	Symptom score decrease	PSA decrease	Prostate volume decrease (%)	Qmax increase	Durability (months)
Maria et al.	Randomized N=30 200 U	62%	51%	68	90%	12
Brisinda et al.	Open label N=77 200 U	64%	58%	55	92%	30
Kuo et al.	Open label N=10 200 U	NA	NA	30	53%	6
Chuang et al.	Open label N=16 100 U	61%	NA	16	73%	6
Chuang et al.	Open label N=21 100 U	62%	NA	19	70%	12
Chuang et al.	Open label N=20 200 U	73%	NA	17	70%	12
Silva et al.	Open label N=21 200 U	Indwelling cath	24%	40	Indwelling cath	12–18
Crawford et al.	Randomized N=125 100 U, 300 U	38%, 46%	0%	0	25%, 27%	12

61–73% and maximum flow rate increase 53–92%) (Table 7.2) (Brisinda et al. 2009; Chuang et al. 2005; Chuang et al. 2006a; Kuo 2005; Maria et al. 2003; Silva et al. 2009a).

A decrease in prostate size that is known to occur following physical or chemical (i.e., onabotulinumtoxinA) denervation in rats was not observed within this study (Doggweiler et al. 1998; McVary et al. 1994). These results suggest that the mechanism of action of onabotulinumtoxinA to improve lower urinary tract symptoms in men with BPH is multi-factorial and not solely related to its effects on altering parasympathetic or sympathetic neural input. Thus, additional directed investigation into the mechanism of action for onabotulinumtoxinA in prostate tissues is appropriate, particularly in view of clinical evidence in human bladders that onabotulinumtoxinA injection can modulate both the expression of sensory nerve receptors and the release of sensory neurotransmitters and nerve growth factor (Apostolidis et al. 2008; Giannantoni et al. 2006; Liu et al. 2009).

One prospective study evaluated the effect of abobotulinumtoxinA for the treatment of BPH (Nikoobakht et al. 2010). Seventy-two men with BPH (i.e., prostate volume) less than 60 g and lower urinary tract symptoms were injected with between 300 and 600 U of abobotulinumtoxinA. Significant reductions in symptom scores, PSA, and residual urine volume and significant increases in maximum flow rate were noted at 6 months of follow-up. No serious complications were noted.

7.6.2 Prostatitis/Prostatodynia

Case Study 7.2: Refractory prostatitis
A 44-year-old divorced male presents with a 2-year history of urinary frequency, urgency, weak stream with straining to void, and pain at the tip of his penis. The patient's symptoms are worse with prolonged sitting and he also describes painful and weak ejaculation. His chronic and debilitating symptoms are interfering with his ability to establish and maintain new relationships. He has seen multiple urologists who have diagnosed him with chronic prostatitis and treated him with non-steroidal analgesics, long-term antibiotics, alpha blockers, neuropathic analgesics (i.e., gabapentin), and prostatic massages without improvement. His last urologist offered him a minimally invasive transurethral prostate microwave therapy procedure but the patient is concerned about the potential for worsening his irritative symptoms and the possibility of developing retrograde ejaculation. The patient desired a second opinion on his condition and, in particular, regarding the possibility of BoNT prostate injection.

Pertinent Exam and Evaluation: On physical exam, the patient had mild prostate enlargement (i.e., 30–35 g, no nodules) but with exquisite tenderness felt in the tip of the penis with palpation of his prostatic apex. Pre- and post-prostatic massage urine and post-massage prostatic fluid were all without evidence of bacterial infection or inflammation. During uroflow studies the patient voided 180 mL with a maximum flow rate of 12 mL/s and a prolonged uroflow with some strain pattern observed (residual urine volume = 0 mL).

Treatment: The known risks were explained to the patient and informed consent was obtained. He was also informed of the two step process requiring that he first undergo local anesthetic block to determine if he would be an appropriate candidate for onabotulinumtoxinA injection. The patient received prophylactic antibiotics and was prepped for transrectal ultrasound-guided prostate injection. Lidocaine jelly was injected into the patient's rectum as a local anesthetic. One percent lidocaine anesthetic was injected in 1 mL aliquots directed at the prostate apex near its junction with the external urethral sphincter. During the injection, the patient noted pain at the tip of his penis. The patient was contacted several hours later and noted a significant (>50%) reduction in his pain symptoms that lasted approximately 4 h. On day 2, the patient returned to for BoNT injection. Under transrectal ultrasound guidance, 100 U of onabotulinumtoxinA diluted in 2 mL of preservative free saline was injected in two injections (i.e., 50 U per injection) at the prostatomembranous junction.

Outcome: Within 4 days, the patient noted an improvement in his urinary stream as well as a decrease in his frequency and urgency. By 1 week after injection, his pain symptoms began dissipating. At 1 month follow-up, the patient was able to stop his daily dose of narcotic analgesics and only require them for "break through pain." The patient's sexual function improved with a more forceful and painless ejaculation. He was restarted on oral gabapentin and at 6 months follow-up described only occasional "flare-ups."

Two small series document results using BoNT to treat voiding dysfunction resulting from non-bacterial prostatitis. In both cases, patients' pain and incomplete emptying symptoms were thought to be related to spastic external urethral sphincters. In one series of four patients, 30 U of onabotulinumtoxinA was injected transperineally targeting the prostatic apex (Maria et al. 1998). Voiding symptoms improved in all 4 patients within 1 week. Moreover, no relapse occurred in 3 out of 4 patients when followed up for a mean of 12 months. Zermann and colleagues injected 200 U of onabotulinumtoxinA into the external urethral sphincter of 11 patients with chronic prostatic pain (Zermann et al. 2000). At 2–4 week follow-up, all patients had a significant reduction in prostatic pain and urethral hypersensitivity as well as objective improvements in residual urine volume and urinary flow rate.

One area we have had anecdotal success is the use of onabotulinumtoxinA as a rescue treatment for penile/urethral pain resulting from a prior prostate surgical procedure (i.e., transurethral microwave therapy, laser prostatectomy, etc.) for BPH. These patients have been refractory to other interventions (i.e., alpha blockers, neuropathic analgesics, biofeedback, etc.). Several patients have been successfully treated with transrectal or transperineal injection of onabotulinumtoxinA (100–200 U) following a positive local block. The improvement in quality of life can be dramatic with reducing or eliminating their chronic source of lower urinary tract pain. Digital rectal exam can often provoke the source of penile or urethral pain with either prostate or external urethral sphincter/levator ani palpation.

7.6.3 Adverse Events

There are little adverse events reported in the literature secondary to prostate BoNT injection. This is opposed to bladder BoNT injection where urinary retention or increased residual urine volume is an anticipated but undesired adverse event or following sphincter BoNT injection where stress urinary incontinence may occur. In our hands, we have found prostate BoNT injection easy to perform and devoid of side effects.

The doses used in intraprostatic injection of BoNT are well below the estimated fatal dose. In addition, all precautions are taken to prevent systemic exposure by using the lowest effective dose and avoiding direct intravascular injection. Dysuria and occasional minor hematuria and epididymitis have been reported (Oeconomou et al. 2008).

The use of prostate BoNT is currently an off-label application of the toxin. Some risks that have been previously reported include temporary urinary retention thought not to be a direct effect of BoNT but due to the large volume injected. Initially, investigators discussed injecting a solution that was 20% of the prostate volume. The rationale for this paradigm was to inject enough of the solution to allow entire gland distribution and to normalize the BoNT effect over different prostate volumes. Unfortunately, a number of men developed temporary overnight retention when a 20% volume was injected. We can image that 16 mL of saline with 200 U onabotulinumtoxinA may cause enough prostate swelling in a man with moderate-severe obstruction and an 80 g prostate to prevent bladder emptying. We have always found excellent distribution of BoNT solution without any retention issues under real time transrectal ultrasound-prostate and have always used 4 mL as our volume of injection without needing adjustments for prostate size.

Additional risks include those specific to ultrasound guided prostate biopsy such as hematuria, hematospermia, hematochezia, and infection. We use the same preparation and antibiotic coverage for our prostate BoNT injection men as we do for transrectal prostate ultrasound and prostate biopsy.

7.7 Conclusions

Because the use of BoNT in prostate is currently "off-label" and not approved by most international regulatory agencies, it should be used with caution until larger randomized clinical trials are completed.

Caution: Given the shorter history of prostate BoNT therapy, the case for recommending BoNT to treat prostate disease is not as strong as for bladder applications. The initial hope of significant shrinking of prostate volume and decreasing PSA are not supported by most recent studies. The improvements with lower urinary tract symptoms appear to equate with symptom reductions described with other minimally invasive techniques. Efficacy lasting 1 year duration has been noted by several reports and this would be highly desirable by most men. Definitive proof of the efficacy of BoNT in the long-term management of BPH remains to be established. There is a paucity of levels I-II studies and the procedure is currently in registry trial and remains an off-label use in selective men with lower urinary tract symptoms refractory to standard oral therapies.

Promise: Despite the cautionary note, the concept of using BoNT prostate treatment is truly exciting although the mechanism of action remains elusive. Prostate BoNT injection is a simple office-based procedure that takes just a few minutes to perform but that can markedly improve patients urinary symptoms for a significant duration (i.e., 1 year) without appreciable local (i.e., retrograde ejaculation) or systemic side effects. In our hands some of the happiest patients who have requested botulinum toxin therapy have been men with either refractory chronic BPH or prostatodynia.

References

Apostolidis A, Jacques TS, Freeman A, Kalsi V, Popat R, Gonzales G, Datta SN, Ghazi-Noori S, Elneil S, Dasgupta P, Fowler CJ (2008) Histological changes in the urothelium and suburothelium of human overactive bladder following intradetrusor injections of botulinum neurotoxin type A for the treatment of neurogenic or idiopathic detrusor overactivity. Eur Urol 53(6):1245–1253

Benaim EA, Montoya JD, Saboorian MH, Litwiller S, Roehrborn CG (1998) Characterization of prostate size, PSA and endocrine profiles in patients with spinal cord injuries. Prostate Cancer Prostatic Dis 1(5):250–255

References

Brisinda G, Cadeddu F, Vanella S, Mazzeo P, Marniga G, Maria G (2009) Relief by botulinum toxin of lower urinary tract symptoms owing to benign prostatic hyperplasia: early and long-term results. Urology 73(1):90–94

Chancellor MB, Fowler CJ, Apostolidis A, de Groat WC, Smith CP, Somogyi GT, Aoki KR (2008) Drug insight: biological effects of botulinum toxin A in the lower urinary tract. Nat Clin Pract Urol 5(6):319–328

Chuang YC, Chiang PH, Huang CC, Yoshimura N, Chancellor MB (2005) Botulinum toxin type A improves benign prostatic hyperplasia symptoms in patients with small prostates. Urology 66(4):775–779

Chuang YC, Chiang PH, Yoshimura N, De Miguel F, Chancellor MB (2006a) Sustained beneficial effects of intraprostatic botulinum toxin type A on lower urinary tract symptoms and quality of life in men with benign prostatic hyperplasia. BJU Int 98(5):1033–1037; discussion 1337

Chuang YC, Huang CC, Kang HY, Chiang PH, Demiguel F, Yoshimura N, Chancellor MB (2006b) Novel action of botulinum toxin on the stromal and epithelial components of the prostate gland. J Urol 175(3 Pt 1):1158–1163

Chuang YC, Tu CH, Huang CC, Lin HJ, Chiang PH, Yoshimura N, Chancellor MB (2006c) Intraprostatic injection of botulinum toxin type-A relieves bladder outlet obstruction in human and induces prostate apoptosis in dogs. BMC Urol 6:12. doi:doi:10.1186/1471-2490-6-12

Chuang YC, Yoshimura N, Huang CC, Wu M, Chiang PH, Chancellor MB (2008) Intraprostatic botulinum toxin a injection inhibits cyclooxygenase-2 expression and suppresses prostatic pain on capsaicin induced prostatitis model in rat. J Urol 180(2):742–748

Doggweiler R, Zermann DH, Ishigooka M, Schmidt RA (1998) Botox-induced prostatic involution. Prostate 37(1):44–50

Giannantoni A, Di Stasi SM, Nardicchi V, Zucchi A, Macchioni L, Bini V, Goracci G, Porena M (2006) Botulinum-A toxin injections into the detrusor muscle decrease nerve growth factor bladder tissue levels in patients with neurogenic detrusor overactivity. J Urol 175(6): 2341–2344

Gormley GJ, Stoner E, Bruskewitz RC, Imperato-McGinley J, Walsh PC, McConnell JD, Andriole GL, Geller J, Bracken BR, Tenover JS, Vaughan ED, Pappas F, Taylor A, Binkowitz B, Ng J (2002) The effect of finasteride in men with benign prostatic hyperplasia. J Urol 167(2 Pt 2):1102–1107; discussion 1108

Kuo HC (2005) Prostate botulinum A toxin injection–an alternative treatment for benign prostatic obstruction in poor surgical candidates. Urology 65(4):670–674

Lepor H, Baumann M, Shapiro E (1987) Identification and characterization of alpha 1 adrenergic receptors in the canine prostate using [125I]-Heat. J Urol 138(5):1336–1339

Liu HT, Chancellor MB, Kuo HC (2009) Urinary nerve growth factor levels are elevated in patients with detrusor overactivity and decreased in responders to detrusor botulinum toxin-A injection. Eur Urol 56(4):700–706

Maria G, Destito A, Lacquaniti S, Bentivoglio AR, Brisinda G, Albanese A (1998) Relief by botulinum toxin of voiding dysfunction due to prostatitis. Lancet 352(9128):625

Maria G, Brisinda G, Civello IM, Bentivoglio AR, Sganga G, Albanese A (2003) Relief by botulinum toxin of voiding dysfunction due to benign prostatic hyperplasia: results of a randomized, placebo-controlled study. Urology 62(2):259–264; discussion 264–265

McVary KT (2006) BPH: epidemiology and comorbidities. Am J Manag Care 12(5 Suppl):S122–S128

McVary KT, Razzaq A, Lee C, Venegas MF, Rademaker A, McKenna KE (1994) Growth of the rat prostate gland is facilitated by the autonomic nervous system. Biol Reprod 51(1):99–107

McVary K, Crawford D, Donnel R, Drews K, Kaplan S, Kusek J, Roehborn C, Bruskewitz R (2010) MIST_2: baseline PSA and total prostate volume predicts clinical response to intraprostatic injection of botulinum toxin for the treatment of LUTS. J Urol 183(suppl):690

Nickel JC, Sander S, Moon TD (2008) A meta-analysis of the vascular-related safety profile and efficacy of alpha-adrenergic blockers for symptoms related to benign prostatic hyperplasia. Int J Clin Pract 62(10):1547–1559

Nikoobakht M, Daneshpajooh A, Ahmadi H, Namdari F, Rezaeidanesh M, Amini S, Pourmand G (2010) Intraprostatic botulinum toxin type A injection for the treatment of benign prostatic hyperplasia: initial experience with Dysport. Scand J Urol Nephrol 44(3):151–157

Oeconomou A, Madersbacher H, Kiss G, Berger TJ, Melekos M, Rehder P (2008) Is botulinum neurotoxin type A (BoNT-A) a novel therapy for lower urinary tract symptoms due to benign prostatic enlargement? A review of the literature. Eur Urol 54(4):765–775

Silva J, Pinto R, Carvalho T, Botelho F, Silva P, Oliveira R, Silva C, Cruz F, Dinis P (2009a) Intraprostatic botulinum toxin type A injection in patients with benign prostatic enlargement: duration of the effect of a single treatment. BMC Urol 9:9

Silva J, Pinto R, Carvallho T, Coelho A, Avelino A, Dinis P, Cruz F (2009b) Mechanisms of prostate atrophy after glandular botulinum neurotoxin type a injection: an experimental study in the rat. Eur Urol 56(1):134–140

Smith CP (2009) Botulinum toxin in the treatment of OAB, BPH, and IC. Toxicon 54(5):639–646

Verhamme KM, Dieleman JP, Bleumink GS, Bosch JL, Stricker BH, Sturkenboom MC (2003) Treatment strategies, patterns of drug use and treatment discontinuation in men with LUTS suggestive of benign prostatic hyperplasia: the Triumph project. Eur Urol 44(5):539–545

Wei JT, Calhoun E, Jacobsen SJ (2005) Urologic diseases in America project: benign prostatic hyperplasia. J Urol 173(4):1256–1261

Zermann D, Ishigooka M, Schubert J, Schmidt RA (2000) Perisphincteric injection of botulinum toxin type A. A treatment option for patients with chronic prostatic pain? Eur Urol 38(4):393–399

Sphincter and Pelvic Floor Disorders Applications

8.1 Introduction

The first indication of BoNT utility in urology was actually not for the overactive bladder but rather injection into the urethral sphincter in spinal cord injured patients to treat detrusor-sphincter dyssynergia (DSD) (Dykstra et al. 1988). In this chapter, we will focus on BoNT injection into the urethral sphincter and pelvic floor for patients with neurogenic detrusor-sphincter dyssynergia, non-neurogenic sphincter discoordination such as dysfunctional voiding or shy bladder syndrome, and pelvic floor spasticity and pain. Because the number of patients who may be candidates for sphincter or pelvic floor injection are small, and etiology and diagnoses diverse, there are no current registry trials to seek regulatory approval for sphincter BoNT application in most developed countries. Therefore, clinicians should be aware that sphincter BoNT injections are off-label applications of BoNT.

8.1.1 Detrusor-Sphincter Dyssynergia Pathology

Normal micturition is based on synergy between a functional bladder and a competent urethral sphincter. The bladder must function to store and empty urine properly, and the neural control resides in the pons and the suprapontine regions of the brain stem to switch between these two modes efficiently and appropriately (Fig. 8.1). Urethral relaxation followed by detrusor contraction is controlled by both autonomic (S2-S4 parasympathetic and T10-L2 sympathetic) and somatic (S2-S4 pudendal) nerves and results in normal coordinated voiding. Neurogenic detrusor overactivity (NDO) typically occurs in upper motor neuron diseases or in injuries with lesions above the sacral spinal cord. For those patients with spinal cord lesions, DSD or uncoordinated micturition between the bladder and sphincter may occur. Patients with pelvic floor spasticity and dysfunction do not have true neurogenic DSD but they are not able to relax their sphincter and pelvic floor during attempted voiding. Both conditions can result in incomplete bladder emptying, high voiding pressure, infection, and vesicoureteral reflux (Fig. 8.2).

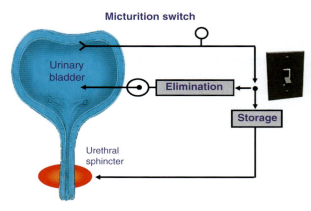

Fig. 8.1 Diagram demonstrating a simplistic view of bladder function. For most of the time, the bladder functions to store urine at low pressures. When one develops a strong desire to void and it is socially acceptable, a "switch" flips and the bladder contracts and expels its contents. Once empty, the bladder switch returns back to the storage mode

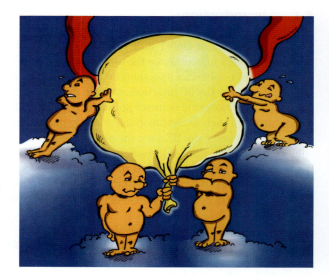

Fig. 8.2 Cartoon comically illustrating the simultaneous overactive and obstructive voiding pattern observed in patients with neurogenic detrusor overactivity and detrusor sphincter dyssynergia

8.2 Indications

8.2.1 Neurogenic DSD

In neurologically impaired patients, the presence of DSD is one of the leading causes of urologic complications. DSD causes high intravesical storage pressures that can lead to infection, stone formation, and upper urinary tract damage. Although neurogenic DSD always occurs in parallel with NDO, treatment of the overactive bladder by antimuscarinics or BoNT does not resolve sphincter spasticity or improve voiding efficiency. Pharmacotherapy of DSD using oral alpha-adrenergic antagonists and striated muscle relaxants are not universally effective. Although some patients report improvement, there are no compelling studies that support their long-term efficacy in DSD. Indwelling or intermittent catheterization is the most common therapy to circumvent DSD. In men who can wear an external condom catheter, sphincterotomy or sphincter stent placement can be successful surgical treatment options.

Transurethral Sphincterotomy has been used for over 50 years and yet it is still a controversial treatment with a high complication rate of bleeding, erectile dysfunction, and failure rates of up to 40%. Oftentimes, failure is related to incomplete resection requiring repeated treatments. In addition, the effects of surgical sphincterotomy are irreversible. Contact laser sphincterotomy is the current technique of choice of most experts for sphincter ablation and incision.

Endourethral Stents can be considered in selected patients with DSD. In this approach, continence is maintained by the competency of the bladder neck. By the same token, concomitant bladder neck dyssynergia in addition to DSD can prevent effective reduction in detrusor leak point pressure by only placing a stent across the external urethral sphincter. Stent placement can be as effective as conventional sphincterotomy and advantageous in regards to reduced hospital stay and reversibility. Additionally, in selective cases of spinal cord patients with DSD where a long segment of the urethra needs to be treated, a second stent can be deployed after the first stent is epithelialized. Hyperplastic tissue in-growth and migration of a stent away from the membranous urethra have been adverse issues associated with stent management of DSD, thereby limiting its utility to a select group of patients.

8.2.1.1 Rationale for BoNT

The goals of DSD treatment are to lower the intravesical pressure, especially detrusor leak point pressure and to promote bladder emptying such that the upper urinary tracts are protected against the high detrusor pressure. The two most common groups of patients with DSD treated with BoNT are patients with spinal cord injury (SCI) and multiple sclerosis (MS).

Compared to external sphincterotomy or intraurethral stent, BoNT treatment is attractive because the treatment is minimally invasive, easy to perform, carries minimal morbidity, and is reversible. The chemical denervation achieved by BoNT is temporary, which offers an advantage by giving male patients the ability to determine if condom catheter is a reasonable bladder management option. In addition, this treatment option offers to the patient the hope of neurorecovery after SCI and the potential to walk again without a sphincter that is permanently damaged. BoNT also offers the opportunity to partially decrease urethral outlet resistance depending on the dosage chosen for moderate degrees of DSD in men and women with neurological diseases.

8.2.2 Non-neurogenic DSD

Goals for sphincter BoNT injection in non-neurogenic DSD patients such as in those diagnosed with dysfunctional voiding or shy bladder syndrome are similar to those goals with neurogenic DSD. The procedure may be considered to help resolve urinary retention, incomplete emptying, and inhibited micturition.

8.2.3 Pelvic Floor and Pain

A number of experts have reported the use of BoNT injection into the pelvic floor for pelvic pain conditions such as vaginismus and painful levator syndrome. What can be the rationale for pelvic floor BoNT injection? BoNT has demonstrated effectiveness in the treatment of several pain disorders of skeletal muscle spasm including focal dystonia, cervical dystonia/spastic torticollis, spasmodic dysphonia, oromandibular dystonia, temporomandibular disorder, refractory myofascial pain syndrome, and tension- and migraine-type headaches.

Chronic pelvic pain in women is a common symptom with a wide variety of etiologies. Conditions such as vestibulodynia and problems affecting deeper structures such as pelvic floor muscle spasm are difficult to treat and can have significant impacts on the quality of life for the sufferer. Symptoms such as painful intercourse (dyspareunia), painful bowel movements (dyschesia) and exacerbation of menstrual pain (dysmenorrhea) are commonly reported by patients.

By eliminating tonic muscle contraction with BoNT injections, nociceptive responses can be blunted. Peripheral desensitization can result from BoNT-induced inhibition of neurotransmitter release from sensory neurons. BoNT also has been shown to block central glutamate release, thus diminishing excitatory amino acid receptors important to the central windup process and pain perception.

The use of BoNT to treat pain is an exciting area of research and there is scientific rationale for the use of BoNT for pelvic floor associated spasm and pain in women and men. For inflammatory conditions, and in areas where muscle spasm is thought to contribute to pain, BoNT has been tried with promising early results.

8.3 What Is the Work-Up

8.3.1 History and Physical Examination

A thorough history including past medical and surgical history and symptoms related to neurologic injury or disease should be obtained. In addition, a patient's sexual history, fecal continence status, results from a bladder diary, and response to medications should be verified. Functional status, especially hand dexterity is particularly important when planning interventions to manage the bladder. In addition, the social setting and support network available to a patient plays an important role in developing a realistic plan. For males who are considering sphincter denervation with BoNT, the ability to hold and maintain a condom catheter should be assessed preoperatively.

8.3.2 Urodynamic Evaluation

Urodynamic testing plays a pivotal role in evaluating patients with neurogenic bladder. This is an important tool to establish baseline bladder storage pressures

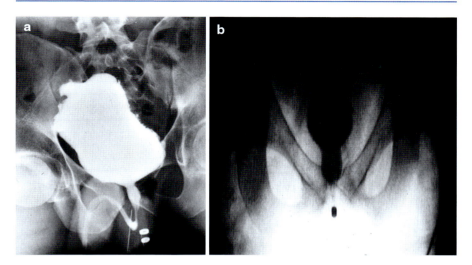

Fig. 8.3 (**a**) Voiding cystourethrogram image demonstrating detrusor-sphincter dyssynergia in a male patient. Note the open bladder neck and prostatic urethral but abrupt cutoff of contrast at level of external urethral sphincter, (**b**) Voiding cystourethrogram image of detrusor sphincter dyssynergia but in a female patient. Note the open bladder neck and proximal urethra but closure at the level of the external sphincter

and behavior that can be useful for diagnosis, prognosis, and management. It is recommended that neurogenic patients undergo serial urodynamic studies as disease processes may change over time. Valuable information such as bladder sensation, filling pressure, detrusor leak point pressure, capacity, compliance, uninhibited detrusor contractions, urine flow rate, urethral pressures, and post-void residual can be achieved with the study. When combined with fluoroscopy, additional data on the mechanics, anatomy, and structure of the bladder and urethra, and the presence of vesicoureteral reflux can be obtained in real time (Fig. 8.3).

The sine qua non of neurogenic DSD diagnosis on urodynamic testing is increased sphincter activity during an involuntary detrusor contraction (Fig. 8.4). Urodynamic diagnosis of dysfunctional voider, shy bladder syndrome, pelvic pain and underactive bladder is often more difficult as patients with pain often have a normal study or lower bladder filling tolerance. Moreover, a dysfunctional voider or person with shy bladder syndrome is likely to have a harder time voiding in the urodynamic laboratory setting such that a voiding phase of the study may not be obtained. Running water, turning down lights, or stepping out of the room are common relaxation methods to aid a patient in being able to void voluntarily. A simple uroflow rate also may be helpful in identifying a dysfunctional voiding pattern (Fig. 8.5).

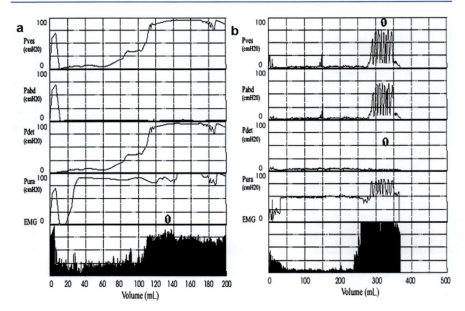

Fig. 8.4 (**a**) Urodynamic image demonstrating elevated electromyographic activity and urethral pressures concurrent with abrupt rise in detrusor pressure in a spinal cord injured patient that is consistent with neurogenic detrusor overactivity and DSD. (**b**) Urodynamic tracing in a non-neurogenic patient that is straining to void. Note elevated Pabd pressures and lack of rise in Pdet pressure that verifies that increase in electromyography signal during void is due to straining and not due to true DSD. *Pves* Intravesical pressure cmH_2O, *Pabd* Intrabdominal pressure cmH_2O, *Pdet* Detrusor pressure (*Pves-Pabd*), *Pure* Intraurethral pressure at the level of the membranous urethra cmH_2O, *CMG* Electromyography

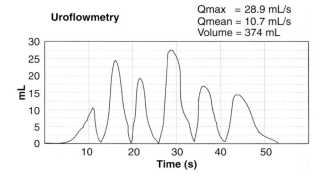

Fig. 8.5 Uroflow rate of non-neurogenic 31-year-old woman with shy bladder syndrome and dysfunctional voiding pattern

8.4 How to Do It

8.4.1 Neurogenic DSD

OnabotulinumtoxinA (Botox®, Allergan, Inc., CA) has been the most commonly used BoNT for the treatment of DSD and pelvic floor conditions. Other serotypes and brands of BoNT should also be effective but doses should be based on the specific toxin used (See chapter on different toxin formulations). We will describe the dose and technique we typically use with sphincter and pelvic floor onabotulinumtoxinA toxin injection in men and women.

BoNT Reconstitution: 100 U of onabotulinumtoxinA are generally utilized in women and 200 U in men. Each 100 U vial of onabotulinumtoxinA is diluted in 2 mL of preservative free saline.

Technique in Men: Male urethral sphincters are injected with a total of 200 U of onabotulinumA diluted in 4 mL of preservative-free saline under local or general anesthesia using a rigid cystoscope loaded with an endoscopic injection needle (e.g., 25-gauge Cook® Williams Needle). OnabotulinumtoxinA is injected in equal aliquots at the 12, 3, 6, and 9 o'clock positions. It is recommended that the injection be directed deeper than urethral bulking agent injections to target the nerve terminals innervating the external (skeletal muscle) sphincter. Other methods described in the literature include perineal and/or transrectal ultrasound guided external urethral sphincter injections (Fig. 8.6) (Chen et al. 2010).

Technique in Women: A 22-gauge short spinal needle is inserted for 1.5 cm at the 3 o'clock and 9 o'clock positions 1 cm lateral to the urethral meatus in the periurethral folds. One millilitre of onabotulinumtoxinA (i.e., 50 U) is injected at each site (Fig. 8.7).

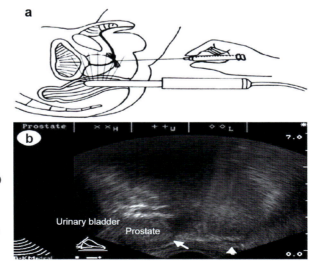

Fig. 8.6 Diagram (**a**) and (**b**) image depicting transrectal ultrasound guided perineal injection of the external urethral sphincter in the male (Copyright obtained from Chen et al. (2010))

Fig. 8.7 Photograph displaying periurethral injection of the external urethral sphincter in the female

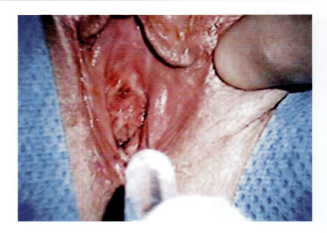

Adequate external urethral sphincter injection should result in a visible reduction in sphincter tone (Fig. 8.8) as well as urodynamic evidence of a decrease in neuromuscular activity via reduced EMG signal.

8.4.2 Simultaneous Bladder and Sphincter BoNT Injection

For selective neurologically impaired patients with both NDO and DSD (i.e., patients with multiple sclerosis), injection of BoNT into the bladder and sphincter may be considered at the same treatment session.

Bladder: Injections with BoNT can be done using either a rigid or flexible cystoscope, under local anesthesia. A total of 100–200 U of onabotulinumA diluted in 10–20 mL of preservative-free saline (i.e., 10 U/mL) are injected submucosally throughout the bladder using an endoscopic injection needle.

Sphincter: Injections of 100 U of onabotulinumA are generally utilized in women and 200 U in men using the techniques described above.

8.4.3 Non-neurogenic DSD

The technique of BoNT injection in non-neurogenic DSD is similar to the technique used for Neurogenic DSD. One additional detail is that non-neurogenic patients often require more local anesthesia and, possibly, general anesthesia. For periurethral injection in women, we have found the liberal use of topical EMLA cream helpful.

We typically use 100 U of onabotulinumtoxinA for patients with underactive bladder who wish to void by abdominal straining, as well as for patients with dysfunctional voiding or poor relaxation of the urethral sphincter. Medications for reduction of urethral resistance such as alpha blockers may be discontinued 1–2 weeks after the BoNT injections if the patient reports clinical improvement.

Fig. 8.8 Cystoscopic images of the male external urethral sphincter in a patient with detrusor sphincter dyssynergia: (**a**) before injection, (**b**) during injection with onabotulinumtoxinA, and (**c**) 1 month after injection (i.e., note lack of coaptation of urethral mucosa demonstrating relaxation of sphincter)

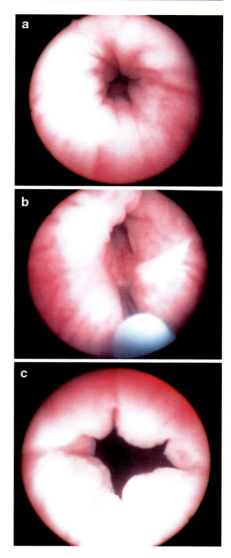

8.4.4 Pelvic Floor and Pain

For the treatment of levator spasm, direct transvaginal injection into the levator muscles can be done. A solution of onabotulinumtoxinA 100–200 U in 4 mL saline is prepared. For levator injections, a disposable pudendal nerve block kit allows for easy transvaginal finger-guided injections of a standardized depth into the pelvic floor muscles. The trocar is guided to the appropriate landmark with the fingertip, the needle is engaged, and the vaginal wall is pierced with the tip of the needle targeting the underlying levator muscles (Fig. 8.9). One millilitre is injected into each

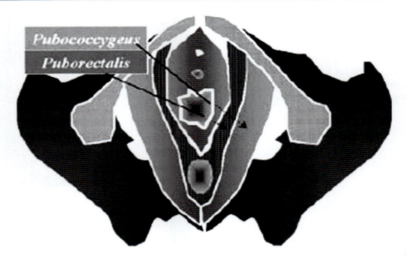

Fig. 8.9 Illustration depicting needle entry point and injection sites for botulinum toxin (*left hand side only represented*) (Copyright obtained from Jarvis et al. (2004))

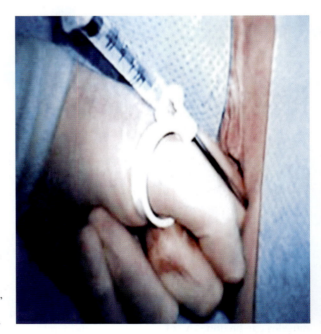

Fig. 8.10 Photograph showing pelvic floor injections using disposable pudendal nerve block trocar and needle. In this photo, the left pubococcygeus muscles are localized medial and distal to the ischial spine and, subsequently, injected with 25 U of onabotulinumtoxinA

of four sites, typically postero-lateral, following aspiration to ensure avoidance of intravascular injection. Proximal injections target the pubococcygeus muscles, at the 5 o'clock and 7 o'clock positions, just medial and distal to the ischial spine

(Fig. 8.10). Distal injections target the puborectalis muscle, at the 5 o'clock and 7 o'clock positions just inside the hymenal ring.

For women with vulvodynia, an injection (i.e., 25–50 U onabotulinumtoxinA) is performed under direct vision targeting superficial perineal muscles using a small gauge spinal needle. Injection sites are placed posterolaterally at the 5 o'clock and 7 o'clock positions within the posterior fourchette and vulva.

8.5 What Are the Results

Case Study 8.1: Multiple Sclerosis (MS) Woman with DSD but who Cannot Self-catheterize

A 52-year-old woman with chronic progressive MS complains of daily incontinence and approximately two urinary tract infections per month. She can void on her own but it takes her a long time in the toilet as she attempts to double void. She now wears adult diapers and has frequent infections needing antibiotics which are exacerbating her MS condition.

Urodynamics: Involuntary detrusor contraction occurred at 265 mL with increased sphincter EMG activity and 215 mL residual urine volume. Urodynamic diagnosis is NDO and DSD.

Previous Management: Oral oxybutynin 15 mg per day, tamsulosin 0.4 mg day, and baclofen 10 mg three times daily without significant improvement. She also tried physical therapy to learn self cathetherization and failed due to poor manual dexterity. She does not want an indwelling catheter or to undergo surgical reconstruction.

BoNT Treatment: The patient understood the off label use of BoNT and its potential risks. She gave informed consent requesting procedure scheduling. The procedure was done in the office with the patient in the lithotomy position. Lidocaine cream was applied to the anterior vagina area for 20 min. Injectable lidocaine 1% 5 mL was used for local anesthesia in the periurethal space using a 28 G needle. 100 U of onabotulinumA was diluted in 2 mL of preservative-free saline and injected at the 3 and 9 o'clock positions periurethrally.

Outcome: After about 4 days, the patient noticed an easier ability to urinate. Post-void residual urine volume decreased after 2 weeks to about 100 mL. She reported spending less time in the bathroom trying to empty her bladder and her incontinence and frequency of urinary tract infection decreased. She continued with her oxybutynin but not the alpha blocker or skeletal muscle relaxant medications. She noticed her improvement lasted about 4–5 months at which point she had more difficulty emptying her bladder and her post-void residual volume increased to over 150 mL. She requested a repeat sphincter injection.

8.5.1 Neurogenic DSD

Dykstra and associates reported the first use of BoNT to treat DSD in 1988. Eleven SCI patients with DSD were injected with 20–240 U of onabotulinumtoxinA into the external sphincter through the perineum or transurethrally with a cystoscope (Dykstra et al. 1988). All 10 patients that were evaluated by electromyography after injection showed signs of sphincter denervation. The maximal urethral pressures in the seven patients in whom they were measured before and after treatment decreased an average of 27 cmH_2O after onabotulinumtoxinA injection. Post-void residual urine volumes decreased by an average of 146 mL after toxin injection in 8 patients. Furthermore, onabotulinumtoxinA decreased autonomic dysreflexia in 5 of 7 patients and the effects of treatment lasted an average of 50 days.

Since Dykstra's initial report, about a dozen peer-reviewed publications have investigated the use of BoNT to treat DSD in SCI and other neurological diseases including its use in pediatric patients. Different toxin formulations, injection dosages, dilution protocols, cumulative dosages, injection frequencies, and injection approaches (cystoscopic vs. transperineal vs. transrectal) have been used in these studies which make comparisons between them difficult. However, most reported clinical improvement in properly selected patients.

Two non-controlled comparative studies demonstrate contradictory results. Chen and Kuo (2004) reported a 41% reduction in intravesical pressures after onabotulinumtoxinA treatment while de Seze and associates (2002) reported no significant change in intravesical pressures following sphincter injections (Chen and Kuo 2004; de Seze et al. 2002). More recently, Smith et al. reported 52 patients with SCI, MS and stroke with significant decreases in maximal voiding pressures and PVR after sphincter onabotulinumtoxinA injection (Smith et al. 2005).

For DSD secondary to multiple sclerosis, the best evidence comes from a multicenter, placebo-controlled, randomized study (Gallien et al. 2005). In that study, a single injection of 100 U of onabotulinumtoxinA via a transperineal approach reduced the intravesical pressure by 21% at 30 days (from 67 to 52 cmH_2O, $p=0.02$). However, treatment neither significantly reduced the post-void residual urine volume or maximal urethral pressures, nor increased the maximal urinary flow rates. These results were less positive than findings reported in SCI patients. The differences in efficacy may represent differences in the pathophysiology of DSD between MS and SCI, or differences in injection techniques (i.e., transperineal injection versus cystoscopic injection).

In a mixed series of 103 patients with voiding dysfunction, performed onabotulinumtoxinA urethral injections using either 50 U ($n=48$) or 100 U ($n=55$). Forty patients (i.e., 39%) had an excellent result, 47 (46%) had significant improvement, and 16 (15%) had treatment failure. Among the patients with an excellent result, patients with detrusor underactivity due to cauda equina lesion (62.5%) or idiopathic cause (61.5%) had the highest success rate, whereas those with DSD (27.6%) ranked last. The overall reported success rate was 84.5%

8.5 What Are the Results

Table 8.1 Sphincter BoNT results

Disease	Number patients	Significant improvement (%)	Moderate improvement (%)	No improvement (%)
Neurologically impaired patients				
1. DSD	29	8 (27.6%)	15 (51.7%)	6 (20.7%)
2. Cauda equine lesion	8	5 (62.5%)	1 (12.5%)	2 (25%)
3. Peripheral neuropathy	14	5 (35.7%)	6 (42.9%)	3 (21.4%)
Patients without neurological diseases				
1. Dysfunctional voiding	20	6 (30%)	14 (70%)	0
2. Non-relaxing urethral sphincter	10	8 (42.1%)	7 (36.8%)	4 (21.1%)
3. Idiopathic detrusor underactivity	13	8 (61.5%)	4 (30.8%)	1 (7.7%)
Total	103	40 (38.8%)	47 (45.7%)	16 (15.5%)

Adapted from Kuo (2003)

(ranged 75–100%). Among the 45 patients presenting with urinary retention, indwelling catheters were removed or clean intermittent catheterization was discontinued in 39 (87%) (Table 8.1). Analysis of the patients with an excellent or improved result shows voiding pressure decreased significantly, as did maximal urethral closure pressure and PVR at 2 or 4 weeks after treatment. The subjective maximum effect was achieved within 1–2 weeks. The mean voiding pressure decreased by 31.8%, maximum flow rate increased by 49.3%, residual urine volume decreased by 60.8% and maximal urethral closure pressure decreased by 28.1%.

Of the studies that have looked specifically at the maximal intravesical pressure, the majority reported reductions in intravesical pressure after BoNT injection (7–41%). Elevated intravesical pressure may be due to persistent obstruction at the bladder neck due to unrecognized detrusor internal sphincter dyssynergia. Reduction of residual urine volume was demonstrated in 7 of 11 studies. The percent improvement of residual urine volume was only 30–54%, so bladder emptying was still incomplete, but the absolute residual volumes were acceptable in most cases (<88 mL). Voiding patterns improved enough that some patients were able to stop intermittent catheterization altogether (5).

Kuo found that 60.6% of 33 patients with neurogenic bladder treated with onabotulinumtoxinA for their DSD were satisfied with their treatment (Kuo 2008). Their relatively low satisfaction rate was somewhat surprising especially given the fact that detrusor pressures and post-void residuals were reduced. The author found that the major reason for dissatisfaction was an increase in urgency and urge incontinence episodes.

8.5.2 Adverse Events

Complications of BoNT injection into the external sphincter are rare and usually self-limiting. Dykstra and Sidi injected 140 U of onabotulinumtoxinA at the first and 240 U at subsequent sessions in the external sphincter of five spinal cord injury patients with DSD (Dykstra et al. 1988). Three patients developed upper extremity weakness that caused difficulty in transferring for 2–3 weeks. This systemic adverse effect was documented by electromyography studies of the deltoid muscle in one of the patients. Appearance of new stress urinary incontinence and exacerbation of preexisting incontinence due to sphincter denervation by BoNT have also been reported. The use of sphincter BoNT is currently an off-label application of the toxin.

Box 8.1: Evidence Based – Detrusor Sphincter Dyssynergia Application

There is one Class I and two Class II studies of BoNT in DSD. In the Class I study, the effects of BoNT vs. placebo were studied on DSD in 86 patients with MS (Gallien et al. 2005). The study employed a single transperineal injection of onabotulinumA, 100 U in 4 mL normal saline, or placebo, into the striated sphincter with EMG guidance. The primary endpoint was the post-void residual urine volume at 30 days. Secondary endpoints included voiding and urodynamic variables. A single injection of BoNT did not decrease residual urine volume in this group of patients with MS. These findings differ from those in patients with SCI and may be due to lower detrusor pressures observed in patients with MS. A small Class II study in five patients with high SCI found BoNT to be superior to placebo for DSD. Measurements of urethral pressure profile, post-voiding residual urine volume and bladder pressure during voiding all decreased in treated patients while no changes from baseline were observed in the placebo group. The duration of the toxin effect averaged 2 months. There was mild generalized weakness lasting 2–3 weeks in three patients after BoNT injections.

Another small Class II study compared the effects of lidocaine (as control) to BoNT in 13 patients with spinal cord disease including traumatic injury, MS, and congenital malformations (de Seze et al. 2002). Measurement of PVR, maximum urethral pressure, maximum detrusor pressure, and micturition diary satisfaction score demonstrated the superiority of BoNT to placebo. No significant side effects were reported in this study.

The American Academy of Neurology recommends BoNT to be considered for DSD but recognizes the limited head-to-head comparisons of treatment options in DSD.

8.5.3 Simultaneous Bladder and Sphincter BoNT Injection

We have experience in 11 patients (3 men and 8 women, mean age 44.6 years old) treated with simultaneous bladder and sphincter BoNT injection. Nine patients had multiple sclerosis and two had thoracic level spinal cord injury. Under sedation anesthesia the patients were injected with onabotulinumtoxinA, 100–200 U in the sphincter (transurethral in men (200 U) and periurethral in women (100 U)) and 200 U in the bladder (Authors personal communication).

Overall mean bladder capacity increased from 205 ± 15 to 324 ± 18 mL ($p < 0.01$) following onabotulinumtoxinA treatment. In 8 out of 11 patients, mean residual urine volume diminished from 155 ± 24 to 100 ± 33 mL. In 3 patients, mean post-void residual urine volume increased from 141 ± 14 to 208 ± 47 mL. While none of the patients developed de novo stress urinary incontinence, one woman's stress incontinence did worsen. Only two patients on clean intermittent catheterization were able to void adequately and stop the self catheterization. Five patients received repeat injections but 3 requested only bladder and 2 requested only sphincter injection.

Our case series experience with simultaneous BoNT into the detrusor and sphincter together was safe and effective in selective patients diagnosed with NDO and DSD who are refractive to standard therapy. The success rate appears to lower when attempting to treat two difficult problems simultaneously than with either bladder or sphincter injection alone.

8.5.4 Non-neurogenic DSD

OnabotulinumA at a dose of 50 U was effective in reducing urethral sphincter resistance among the patients with detrusor underactivity and difficult urination. Of the 4 men and 15 women, 18 (90%) were treated satisfactorily. Among these patients, the mean quality of life score improved, median voiding pressure decreased (56.5 ± 41.2 vs. 39.0 ± 32.1 cmH$_2$O), and residual urine volume decreased (300 ± 189.1 v 50 ± 153.6 mL) 2 weeks after treatment and improvement was maintained for at least 3 months. In 7 patients, the indwelling catheters were removed, and in 4 patients who performed self catheterization, the frequency decreased or it was discontinued. The other 7 patients with difficult urination had significant improvement in their obstructive symptom scores.

In patients with dysfunctional voiding due to urethral sphincter overactivity, non-bacterial prostatitis and detrusor underactivity, BoNT has been shown to have a therapeutic effect in improving voiding efficiency and recovering detrusor contractility in a number of patients with few reported adverse effects. We found that after BoNT injection 67% of the patients were able to void smoothly with residual urine volume decreased by 71% and voiding pressure decreased by 38% (Phelan et al. 2001).

Kuo evaluated the effects of onabotulinumtoxinA urethral injection in 27 patients with idiopathic low detrusor contractility (Kuo 2007). Detrusor contractility recovered in 48% of those treated. Patients with normal bladder sensation combined with poor relaxation or hyperactive urethral sphincter activity were most likely to respond to urethral injections with onabotulinumtoxinA. In 38% of patients, the therapeutic effect of restoring detrusor contractility lasted over 1 year.

Case Study 8.2: Dysfunctional Voider Man
A 48-year-old man with a life long history of difficulty voiding in public bathrooms was suspended from his manufacturing job because he was not able to give a urine specimen during a random drug screen. "I could not go when there were two people standing in the bathroom with me". He has had several episodes in his life of not being able to void and having to go to the emergency room for catheterization. He tried alpha blocker, biofeedback and hypnosis without improvement. Previous cystoscopy revealed no urethral stricture and moderate trabeculation. Renal function was normal.

Urodynamics: The patient could not void with the catheter inserted in his penis. His bladder sensation was normal to a capacity of 370 mL with normal compliance. Free uroflow with EMG after filling demonstrated an intermittent voiding pattern with increased EMG signal but no residual urine volume.

BoNT Treatment: After informed consent for off label use, the procedure was done in the surgical center with brief sedation anesthesia as requested by the patient. A rigid cystoscope was used with a 25 G endoscopic needle for injection. 200 U of onabotulinumA diluted in 4 mL of preservative-free saline was injected deeply into four sites in the membranous urethral sphincter (50 U/mL per site). The patient did not require a catheter post-procedure.

Outcome: The patient did not develop stress incontinence, impotence or retrograde ejaculation following injection. He did report significant hesitancy for the first 72 h but was able to void with analgesic and muscle relaxant medications. After 1 week, the patient noticed an easier time to urinate and this improvement persisted over 6 months. Although he still chooses private stalls over public urinals, the patient has noticed a clear cut improvement and reports he is not "fighting himself as much." "My bladder is not as shy as it was" and he was able to give a specimen at work and passed his drug screen.

8.5.5 Post-surgical Retention

Patients after radical hysterectomy for cervical cancer may have difficult urination due to detrusor underactivity and non-relaxing urethral sphincter. Urethral injection of BoNT can be effectively used to treat lower urinary tract dysfunctions in these patients (Kuo 2005). Thirty patients with difficult urination after radical hysterectomy due to cervical cancer were enrolled to receive urethral injection of 100 U of onabotulinumtoxinA ($n = 20$) or medical treatment as controls ($n = 10$). After urethral BoNT injection, 8 patients had excellent results (40%) and 8 had improved results (40%) in the onabotulinumtoxinA group. Both voiding pressure and post-void residual urine volume also showed significant improvement after onabotulinumtoxinA treatment. The maximal effect appeared about 1 week after treatment. The duration of therapeutic effect ranged from 3 to 9 months. Mild stress urinary incontinence and nocturnal enuresis were noted in 7 patients (35%). No significant changes in voiding parameters were noted in the control group.

Postoperative urinary retention following pubovaginal sling procedure has traditionally been thought to be due to surgical edema or bladder neck elevation and urethral compression. Fitzgerald and Brubaker reported on abnormal external urethral sphincter activity as a cause for postoperative voiding difficulty (FitzGerald and Brubaker 2001).

We have demonstrated success with pelvic floor/sphincter onabotulinumtoxinA injection in a patient with post-urethral sling retention and detrusor acontractility (Smith et al. 2002). Presumably, our patient's postoperative retention was not related to anatomical obstruction but due to a hyperactive sphincter as evidenced by her successful response to BoNT injection (i.e., spontaneous voiding with return of detrusor contractility by urodynamics).

8.5.6 Bladder Neck Dyssynergia (Primary Bladder Neck Obstruction)

Lim and Quek evaluated the effects of onabotulinumtoxinA on voiding parameters in 8 men diagnosed by video-urodynamic study and who had failed medical treatment (Lim and Quek 2008). Eight patients with bladder-neck dyssynergia had 100 U of onabotulinumtoxinA injected transurethrally into the bladder neck and proximal prostatic urethra laterally (10 U/mL × 10 sites). At 6 weeks, 7 of 8 (87.5%) patients had >50% reduction of international prostate symptom scores from baseline. Six of eight (75.0%) patients had >3 mL/s increase in peak urinary flow rate with overall mean peak urinary flow rates improving from 11.6 to 17.2 ($p = 0.048$) at 6 weeks. Micturition frequency decreased 46% and quality of life component of the international prostate symptom scores improved 47%. Symptom relief lasted 6 months to over 1 year. No patient reported any adverse effects or ejaculation dysfunction.

Bladder neck or sphincter injections with onabotulinumtoxinA may also be considered as a tool to differentiate the source of obstruction in unclear cases as well as to predict the response to definitive and irreversible treatments.

8.5.7 Pelvic Floor and Pain

Botulinum toxin injection of the pubococcygeus and puborectalis muscles was reported in 12 women with chronic pelvic pain and pelvic floor muscle hypertonicity (Jarvis et al. 2004). OnabotulinumA 40 U was injected transvaginally into the puborectalis and pubococcygeus bilaterally in a total of four sites, using three different concentrations of onabotulinumtoxinA (10, 20, and 100 U/mL). At 12 weeks follow-up, significant pain reduction scores for dyspareunia and dysmenorrhea, improvements in sexual activity scores, and improvements in bladder function scores were observed.

Pain caused by spasm of the pelvic floor can be a difficult condition to treat. Ghazizadeh and Nikzad injected 150–400 U of abobotulinumtoxinA (Dysport®) into the levator ani of 24 women with refractory vaginismus. Symptoms significantly improved such that 75% of patients were able to have satisfactory intercourse. The results of these initial studies are encouraging (Ghazizadeh and Nikzad 2004).

In contrast, a double blind randomized clinical trial of onabotulinumtoxinA vs. saline, 60 patients with 2 years or more of chronic pelvic pain received either onabotulinumtoxinA 80 U (20 U/mL) or normal saline injections into the puborectalis and pubococcygeus muscles (Abbott et al. 2006). After 26 weeks of follow-up, quality of life measures were improved in both BoNT and placebo groups, but the difference between BoNT and placebo groups did not reach statistical significance. However, pelvic floor pressure was reduced with BoNT compared to placebo. The investigators concluded that the lack of significant superiority of BoNT in quality of life improvements was related to the relatively small study size and imperfect quality of life assessment tools.

8.5.8 Pain Due to Hypertonic Pelvic Floor Muscles

Romito and associates (2004) evaluated BoNT injections on hypertonic pelvic floor muscles of patients suffering from genital pain syndromes (Romito et al. 2004). They report two cases of women complaining of a genital pain syndrome resistant to pharmacological therapies and rehabilitation exercises associated with a documented involuntary tonic contraction of the levator ani muscle as a defense reaction triggered by vulvar pain.

Romito and associates performed BoNT injections into the levator ani with the intent to relieve pelvic muscular spasms. Within 1 week of the injections, both patients reported a complete resolution of painful symptomatology, lasting for several months. The authors concluded that BoNT injections are indicated in patients with genital pain syndrome with documented pelvic muscle hyperactivity, whose

> **Case Study 8.3: Woman with Pelvic Pain**
> A 34-year-old married woman with chronic pelvic pain who is currently attending graduate school. Her pain is localized to her pelvic floor and perineum. It is worse with prolonged sitting and is severe enough that she can no longer have sexual intercourse with her husband. She has tried pelvic floor therapy with limited improvement. While valium provides some relief, it interferes with her school performance.

> Physical Exam: On pelvic exam, the patient is found to have exquisite tenderness and increased tone within her levator ani muscles. On palpation, her pain radiates to her vulvar area and perineum.
>
> BoNT Treatment: After informed consent for off-label use, the procedure is performed in the surgical center with brief sedation anesthesia per patient request. Following lidocaine cream intravaginal anesthetic, a pudendal nerve block kit is used for targeted onabotulinumtoxinA delivery. A total of 100 U of onabotulinumtoxinA diluted in 2 mL of preservative-free saline was injected at the 5 o'clock and 7 o'clock positions in the pubococcygeus and puborectalis muscles for a total of four injections. Gauze pressure was applied for hemostasis.
>
> Outcome: Within 3–4 days, the patient noted a significant reduction in pelvic floor and perineal pain. She was now able to tolerate sitting through a full schedule of classes at school. In addition, she has become sexually active with her husband and reports a marked improvement in their relationship. While she describes mild pelvic discomfort the day following intercourse, it is transient and minor in severity compared to before treatment.

symptoms arise not only from genital inflammation and lesions, but also, and sometimes chiefly, from levator ani myalgia.

8.5.9 Vulvodynia

Application of BoNT for vulvodynia has also been reported. Gunter and associates (2004) reported a case of refractory vulvodynia with severe dyspareunia successfully managed with BoNT injection (Gunter et al. 2004). There is limited data, in the form of case reports and small series, to indicate that BoNT used in the vulva may have a benefit for 3–6 months after injection of 20–40 U of OnabotulinumA for women with provoked vestibulodynia (Abbott 2009). Re-treatment is reported to be successful and side effects are limited. Controlled studies are essential to further explore this indication.

In summary, BoNT treatment for a variety of gynecological indications seems successful with limited side effects, although there are minimal data, particularly in superficial, non-muscular conditions such as vulvodynia. We believe more research is needed before we can make broader recommendation. Physical therapy could be used as a non-invasive first-line treatment, with BoNT injections reserved for those who are refractory to treatment.

8.5.10 Chronic Prostatitis/Male Chronic Pelvic Pain Syndrome

Only one clinical study has specifically addressed the use of BoNT for the treatment of male chronic pelvic pain (Zermann et al. 2000). Eleven men with chronic prostatic pain of greater than 12 months duration, aged 32–66 years were studied. OnabotulinumA 200 U was administered by transurethral perisphincteric injection under direct vision using a 22 gauge needle via 3–4 injection sites. At 2–4 weeks follow-up, 9 of 11 patients reported subjective improvement. Visual pain scores decreased from 7.2 to 1.6. Significant decreases in pelvic floor tenderness, functional urethral length, urethral closure pressure, residual urine volume, and increases in average and maximal uroflow were observed. No other problems were reported except for one patient developing stress urinary incontinence after BoNT injection.

8.6 Conclusion

We would like to finish this chapter on a cautionary note: the case for BoNT in sphincter and pelvic floor applications are based on outside registry trials and rely on expert opinions. Despite promising findings regarding the use of BoNT to treat chronic genitourinary pain syndromes, a standardization of terminology, technique and prospective randomized trials with standardized outcome measures in order to fully evaluate the clinical effectiveness of this promising modality is needed.

Functional electrical stimulation is a valuable tool used in various medical fields to induce muscle activation, walking, and even bladder control. For the bladder, modulation and stimulation of sacral nerve roots can provide an alternative treatment option in patients with voiding dysfunction and chronic pelvic pain. We believe the future holds great excitement and promise with local introduction of botulinum toxin to biologically modulate the sphincter as an alternative to, or in combination with electrical neuromodulation to help restore normal voluntary micturition while reducing painful stimuli.

References

Abbott J (2009) The use of botulinum toxin in the pelvic floor for women with chronic pelvic pain- a new answer to old problems? J Minim Invasive Gynecol 16:130–135

Abbott JA, Jarvis SK, Lyons SD, Thomson A, Vancaille TG (2006) Botulinum toxin type A for chronic pain and pelvic floor spasm in women: a randomized controlled trial. Obstet Gynecol 108:915–923

Chen YH, Kuo HC (2004) Botulinum A toxin treatment of urethral sphincter pseudodyssynergia in patients with cerebrovascular accidents or intracranial lesions. Urol Int 73:156–161; discussion 161–162

Chen SL, Bih LI, Chen GD, Huang YH, You YH, Lew HL (2010) Transrectal ultrasound-guided transperineal botulinum toxin a injection to the external urethral sphincter for treatment of detrusor external sphincter dyssynergia in patients with spinal cord injury. Arch Phys Med Rehabil 91:340–344

de Seze M, Petit H, Gallien P, de Seze MP, Joseph PA, Mazaux JM, Barat M (2002) Botulinum a toxin and detrusor sphincter dyssynergia: a double-blind lidocaine-controlled study in 13 patients with spinal cord disease. Eur Urol 42:56–62

Dykstra DD, Sidi AA, Scott AB, Pagel JM, Goldish GD (1988) Effects of botulinum A toxin on detrusor-sphincter dyssynergia in spinal cord injury patients. J Urol 139:919–922

FitzGerald MP, Brubaker L (2001) The etiology of urinary retention after surgery for genuine stress incontinence. Neurourol Urodyn 20:13–21

Gallien P, Reymann JM, Amarenco G, Nicolas B, de Seze M, Bellissant E (2005) Placebo controlled, randomised, double blind study of the effects of botulinum A toxin on detrusor sphincter dyssynergia in multiple sclerosis patients. J Neurol Neurosurg Psychiatry 76:1670–1676

Ghazizadeh S, Nikzad M (2004) Botulinum toxin in the treatment of refractory vaginismus. Obstet Gynecol 104:922–925

Gunter J, Brewer A, Tawfik O (2004) Botulinum toxin a for vulvodynia: a case report. J Pain 5:238–240

Jarvis SK, Abbott JA, Lenart MB, Steensma A, Vancaillie TG (2004) Pilot study of botulinum toxin type A in the treatment of chronic pelvic pain associated with spasm of the levator ani muscles. Aust N Z J Obstet Gynaecol 44:46–50

Kuo HC (2005) Effectiveness of urethral injection of botulinum A toxin in the treatment of voiding dysfunction after radical hysterectomy. Urol Int 75:247–251

Kuo HC (2007) Recovery of detrusor function after urethral botulinum A toxin injection in patients with idiopathic low detrusor contractility and voiding dysfunction. Urology 69:57–61; discussion 61–62

Kuo HC (2008) Satisfaction with urethral injection of botulinum toxin A for detrusor sphincter dyssynergia in patients with spinal cord lesion. Neurourol Urodyn 27:793–796

Lim SK, Quek PL (2008) Intraprostatic and bladder-neck injection of botulinum A toxin in treatment of males with bladder-neck dyssynergia: a pilot study. Eur Urol 53:620–625

Phelan MW, Franks M, Somogyi GT, Yokoyama T, Fraser MO, Lavelle JP, Yoshimura N, Chancellor MB (2001) Botulinum toxin urethral sphincter injection to restore bladder emptying in men and women with voiding dysfunction. J Urol 165:1107–1110

Romito S, Bottanelli M, Pellegrini M, Vicentini S, Rizzuto N, Bertolasi L (2004) Botulinum toxin for the treatment of genital pain syndromes. Gynecol Obstet Invest 58:164–167

Smith CP, O'Leary M, Erickson J, Somogyi GT, Chancellor MB (2002) Botulinum toxin urethral sphincter injection resolves urinary retention after pubovaginal sling operation. Int Urogynecol J Pelvic Floor Dysfunct 13:185–186

Smith CP, Nishiguchi J, O'Leary M, Yoshimura N, Chancellor MB (2005) Single-institution experience in 110 patients with botulinum toxin A injection into bladder or urethra. Urology 65:37–41

Zermann D, Ishigooka M, Schubert J, Schmidt RA (2000) Perisphincteric injection of botulinum toxin type A. A treatment option for patients with chronic prostatic pain? Eur Urol 38:393–399

Part IV
Role of BoNT in Medicine

Non-urological Uses of Toxin with Genitourinary Insight

9.1 Introduction

Since botulinum neurotoxin was initially approved for clinical use by the USA Food and Drug Administration in 1989, it has become a powerful therapeutic tool in the treatment of a variety of neurologic, ophthalmic, and other disorders manifested by abnormal, excessive, or inappropriate muscle contractions. Now, botulinum toxin (BoNT) has received approval from international regulatory agencies for uses including blepharospasm, strabismus, a other facial nerve disorders, cervical dystonia, hyperhidrosis, and cosmetic disorders. BoNT has also been applied in the clinical management of pain in a number of areas, including myofascial pain disorders, low back pain, and was recently approved for the prevention of recurrent migraine headaches. For the clinician interested in the genitourinary application of BoNT, an evaluation of some interesting uses of BoNT in other fields may offer insight and a fresh perspective (Table 9.1).

9.2 BoNT in Pain Syndromes

9.2.1 Back Pain

Probably every one of us has either experienced or knows someone with chronic low back pain. It is a common problem and back or spine problems account for 16.5% of all disability in the United States.

Although chronic pain's mechanism of action is complex, hypothesized mechanisms for the pain are based on:
1. An increase in pain fiber density
2. An increase in neuropeptide release, which further exacerbates the inflammatory reaction
3. Sensitization by neuropeptides of nerves that convey pain signals

BoNT can relax the injected muscles and also modulate these pain-signaling pathways(Aoki 2003; Difazio and Jabbari 2002).

Table 9.1 BoNT in other fields and relevance to genitourinary system

Nonurological application	Mechanism of interest	Genitourinary implications
Pain	Muscle spasticity and sensory neuromodulation	Bladder pain
		Prostatitis
		Pelvic floor pain; trigger points
Hyperhidrosis	Activity on glands	Benign prostate hyperplasia
		Vulvar vestibulitis
Gastrointestinal tract	Activity on smooth muscle	Bladder
		Bladder neck, vagina

9.2.1.1 Efficacy of BoNT in Managing Chronic Back Pain

One randomized, controlled trial evaluated the efficacy of onabotulinumtoxinA (40 U/site at five lumbar paravertebral levels on the side of maximum discomfort) or placebo in 31 patients with chronic low back pain (Foster et al. 2001). At 3 and 8 weeks postinjection, back pain was reduced by >50% in a significantly greater proportion of onabotulinumtoxinA-treated patients (73.3% and 60% at 3 and 8 weeks, respectively; $P \leq 0.01$) compared with placebo-treated patients (2.5% and 12.5%). Disability resulting from back pain also improved in more onabotulinumtoxinA-treated patients (66.7%) compared with placebo (18.8%; $P=0.011$).

An unblinded open-label study of 20 patients with piriformis syndrome in which subjects were treated either unilaterally or bilaterally with 5,000 units of rimabotulinumtoxinB found significant reduction in mean visual analog scale scores for buttock and hip pain at weeks 4, 12, and 16 and for low back pain at weeks 2, 12, and 16 after treatment (Lang 2004). Most reports suggest that BoNT therapy for back pain is safe and effective and provides local relief directly at the site of pain or injury without causing systemic side effects.

9.2.2 Myofascial Pain Syndromes

Myofascial pain syndrome is an acute or chronic pain disorder of soft tissue, frequently associated with sensory or motor autonomic symptoms, that is referred from active myofascial trigger points. A trigger point is a palpable knot or mass in a taut band of muscle (usually 3–6 mm in diameter), associated with tenderness and referred pain into well-defined areas remote from the trigger point area. Although the mechanisms that precipitate the pain in these syndromes vary, it is likely that a central mechanism contributes to many complex pain syndromes (Smith et al. 2002a).

The precise incidence of myofascial pain syndrome is unknown but it is one of the most common painful conditions among the general population, accounting for 30–85% of patients seen in pain clinics (Han and Harrison 1997). Current treatment options for patients with myofascial pain syndrome are listed in Table 9.2.

Table 9.2 Myofascial pain syndrome: current treatment approaches
- Oral medications
  - Steroidal and nonsteroidal anti-inflammatory drugs
  - Antidepressants
  - Vasodilators
- Injection of local anesthetics or saline
- Spray and stretch
- Physiotherapy

Adapted from Porta (2000) and Smith et al. (2002b)

9.2.2.1 Efficacy of BoNT in Patients with Myofascial Pain Syndrome

BoNT therapy may be considered in soft-tissue syndromes refractory to traditional management with physical therapy, electrical muscle stimulation, and other approaches. BoNT treatment also may be useful as an adjunct that reduces pain sufficiently for patients to resume more conservative therapy. The major benefits of treatment with BoNT are its long duration of action and lack of significant side effects (Smith et al. 2002a).

OnabotulinumtoxinA (BOTOX®) and abobotulinumtoxinA (Myobloc®) have been shown to provide effective relief of pain associated with myofascial pain syndrome, as well as fibromyalgia and other types of soft-tissue syndromes (Porta 2000; Smith et al. 2002a). Treated 33 myofascial pain syndrome patients with 50 or 100 U of BoNT-A or placebo and noted significant changes from baseline in the post treatment assessment at 4 months in all treatment groups, but without significant differences among them. Others studies did not find efficacy using trigger point injection for BoNT treatment of myofascial pain syndrome (Ferrante et al. 2005).

9.2.2.2 Safety of BoNT in Patients with Myofascial Pain Syndrome

In one of the larger studies of onabotulinumtoxinA in 77 patients with myofascial pain syndrome, no side effects were observed in 83.1% of cases. The most frequently reported side effects were numbness at the injection site (6.5%), muscle weakness (2.6%), and flu-like syndrome (2.6%) (De Andres et al. 2003). Overall, side effects were mild and transient.

9.2.2.3 BoNT Injection Method and Dosing for Patients with Myofascial Pain Syndrome

A quick outline of some general concepts in the treatment of myofascial pain syndrome that may be helpful for clinicians considering trigger point approaches in the genitourinary system:
- In deep muscles (iliopsoas, quadratus lumborum, and piriformis), injection should be delivered to a single site.
- The number of injection sites is chosen according to the number of trigger points identified. In each site, 10 units of onabotulinumtoxinA is commonly injected.
- Total dose of onabotulinumtoxinA ranges from 25 to 100 U per treatment session (De Andres et al. 2003).

9.2.3 Headache and Migraine

Of the 45 million Americans affected by headache disorders, an estimated 28 million suffer from migraine (Lipton et al. 2002, 2001). In migraine, nociceptive peptide mediators such as substance P, calcitonin gene-related peptide (CGRP), and neurokinin A are released from perivascular nerve fibers in response to stimulation of the trigeminal nerve (Moskowitz 1993). These mediators trigger the trigemino-vascular system to transmit nociceptive information to the brainstem via the action of glutamate. It has been hypothesized that migraine sufferers have an altered peripheral glutamate homeostasis and persistent neuronal hyperexcitability that predisposes them to the pain associated with a migraine attack (Ramadan 2003).

9.2.3.1 BoNT Headache Mechanism of Action

The mechanisms by which BoNT alleviates headache pain are not fully understood, but they are more complex than simple muscle relaxation resulting from the inhibition of acetylcholine release at the neuromuscular junction. Direct and indirect evidence suggests that distinct antinociceptive effects of BoNT contribute to its observed efficacy in alleviating headache pain. BoNT inhibits release of substance P, CGRP, and glutamate, which are known to be involved in the pain pathways (Aoki 2003). BoNT may prevent central sensitization in wide dynamic range neurons in the trigeminal nucleus caudalis (Fig. 9.1).

9.2.3.2 Efficacy of BoNT in Patients with Headache

Two randomized, controlled trials support the clinical efficacy of BoNT in the treatment of migraine headaches. In one trial, treatment with 25 U of onabotulinumtoxinA reduced the frequency and severity of migraine compared with vehicle treatment and it also reduced the incidence of migraine-associated vomiting and the need for acute migraine medication usage (Silberstein et al. 2000). In a 3-month study, 60 migraine patients were randomly assigned to receive placebo in the frontal and neck muscles, or 16 U of onabotulinumtoxinA in the frontal muscles and placebo in the neck muscles, or a total of 100 U of onabotulinumtoxinA in the frontal and neck muscles. Although accompanying symptoms were significantly reduced in the 16 U but not the 100 U treatment group, no efficacy of onabotulinumtoxinA was found in the prophylactic treatment of migraine (Evers et al. 2004).

9.2.3.3 Safety of BoNT in Patients with Headache

Clinical trials involving over 2,000 headache patients have demonstrated that BoNT injections, as preventive treatment of headache, have been safe and well tolerated, with a notable lack of the systemic effects of other headache medications. BoNT treatment-related side effects such as muscle weakness, injection site pain, headache, rash, bruising, and eyebrow and eyelid ptosis are generally transient and mild to moderate in severity (Blumenfeld et al. 2003; Silberstein et al. 2000; Troost 2004). Minor side effects can be minimized by injection technique (Blumenfeld et al. 2003). Based on limited clinical data, BoNT serotype B treatment for headache

Fig. 9.1 Botulinum toxin blocked glutamate release which decrease C fiber and A delta fiber activation, and sensitization, or up regulation. Peripheral BoNT can inhibit neuron and spinal cord pain response

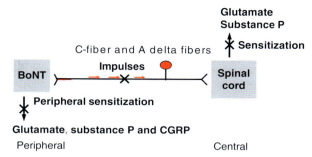

Table 9.3 Headache anatomical injection sites and onabotulinumtoxinA dose

Muscle	OnabotulinumtoxinA units/site	Number of injection sites
Cervical paraspinal muscles	2.5	1–3 per side
Frontalis	2.5	8–12 (4–6 per side)
Occipitalis	2.5–5.0	2 (1 per side)
Sternocleidomastoid	5.0–10.0	2
Temporalis	2.5–5.0	8–10 (4–5 per side)
Trapezius	5.0–10.0	2–6 (1–3 per side)

Adapted from Blumenfeld et al. (2003)

also appears to be well tolerated. Adverse events were minor and included dry mouth and injection-site pain lasting a few days (Opida 2002).

9.2.3.4 Administration of BoNT in Patients with Headache

There are several recommended BoNT injection protocols for headache; these can be described as a fixed-site approach, a follow-the-pain approach, and a combination approach. (Blumenfeld 2003; Blumenfeld et al. 2003). Table 9.3 gives a description of muscle groups and dose per site commonly used by headache experts.
- *Fixed-site* method is often used for patients with migraine or migrainous headache and uses fixed symmetrical injection sites with a range of predetermined doses. Injections should be bilateral.
- *Follow-the-pain* approach adjusts the sites and doses depending on where the patient feels pain and where the examiner can elicit pain and tenderness on palpation of the muscle. For patients with coexisting migraine and tension headaches. Injections may be unilateral or bilateral, depending on signs and symptoms.

9.3 BoNT in the Gastrointestinal Tract

The use of BoNT to relax overactive smooth muscle sphincters has been applied to the therapeutic management of achalasia, chronic anal fissure, gastroparesis, and postcholecystectomy pain syndromes, among others.

9.3.1 Achalasia

Achalasia is a primary esophageal motility disorder associated with impaired relaxation of the lower esophageal sphincter and with dysfunctional or absent peristalsis in the body of the esophagus (Garofalo and Pofahl 2002). The etiology is believed to involve a selective loss of postganglionic inhibitory neurons of the myenteric plexus of the esophagus and lower esophageal sphincter and the persistence of excitatory postganglionic cholinergic neurons. This imbalance in neurotransmitter release accounts for sustained lower esophageal sphincter tone and failure of the lower esophageal sphincter to relax, resulting in a functional obstruction. Common symptoms of achalasia include dysphagia, regurgitation, weight loss, chest pain, and heartburn, and may also include vomiting, reflux, choking, and cough.

Treatment of achalasia is palliative and aimed at reducing lower esophageal sphincter pressure. Options include pharmacologic agents, pneumatic balloon dilatation, intraphincteric botulinum toxin injection, open surgical myotomy, and minimally invasive surgical approaches (Kaufman and Oelschlager 2005).

9.3.1.1 BoNT Clinical Studies in Achalasia

For treatment of achalasia, BoNT is normally injected (usual dose, 100 U onabotulinumtoxinA) during a routine upper endoscopy and adds only a few minutes to a standard diagnostic procedure. In a randomized, double-blind, placebo-controlled trial, patients receiving 80 U of onabotulinumtoxinA had a significant decrease in mean symptom score versus baseline at 1 week, while those receiving placebo did not. All 21 patients were eventually given onabotulinumtoxinA. At 6 months, 14 (74%) were in remission, 11 after a single injection (Pasricha et al. 1995). In a multicenter study of 55 patients, clinical improvement was observed in 75% of patients at 2 weeks. At month 6, clinical improvement was seen in 33 patients, 27 of whom had a single injection (Cuilliere et al. 1997). No serious adverse effects were reported.

Short-term positive response of achalasia to BoNT is noted in over 65% of patients. Single injections may not produce permanent relief and optimal BoNT efficacy may require repeated injections (Friedenberg et al. 2004).

Expert Opinions: Gastrointestinal vs. Genitourinary Effects
Pankaj Jay Pasricha, M.D.
> Professor of Medicine and by courtesy, Surgery
> Chief of the Division of Gastroenterology and Hepatology
> Stanford University School of Medicine

Much has been written about the "wonder-drug" that is botulinum toxin in the scientific literature and the lay press. The therapeutic targets are dizzyingly diverse and include every region of the body, going far beyond the classic skeletal muscle disorders. In 1991, I started experimenting with the use of the toxin for gastrointestinal disorders. At that time, it was not clear whether the toxin could reduce visceral smooth muscle in vivo, even though ileus had long been recognized as part of the syndrome of botulism. After demonstrating proof-of-principle in animal models, we prepared to treat our first human, a patient with achalasia despite significant push-back from colleagues and peers who questioned both the wisdom and effectiveness of such an approach. The rest, as they say, is history, and today, botulinum toxin is widely regarded as safe and effective in reducing the contractility of smooth muscle, contractility of gastrointestinal, urinary and even genital origin.

Beyond the obvious potential benefits to patients, what is not readily appreciated is the use of the toxin to advance our knowledge of both the basic biology of visceral muscle as well as the pathophysiology of related disorders. Thus, through the use of botulinum toxin, we have learned that net cholinergic and other vesicle-based neurotransmitter effects on smooth muscle are excitatory. We have also for the first time understood that in the absence of such neural input, the muscle becomes stunned, rendering it hyposensitive to exogenous agonists, in contrast to skeletal muscle which displays supersensitivity under the same conditions.

An equally important role for this agent may be to help resolve the often-encountered clinical dilemma of whether neurogenically mediated muscle spasm is contributing to the symptoms in a given patient. The pathophysiology of many so-called functional disorders of the gastrointestinal and urogenital tract is obscure, although "muscle spasm" is often suspected. A positive result of the "toxin test" may indeed be the most reliable way of predicting whether more invasive treatments such as surgical ablation of the suspect muscle are justified.

Thus, more than 100 years after he wrote them, Claude Bernard's words still ring true: Poisons can be employed as a means for the destruction of life or as agents for the treatment of the sick, but in addition to these two well recognized uses there is a third of particular interest to the physiologist. For him the poison becomes an instrument which dissociates and analyzes the most delicate phenomena of living structures and by attending carefully to their mechanism in causing death he can learn indirectly much about the physiological processes of life.

9.3.2 Chronic Anal Fissure

Chronic idiopathic anal fissure is a common and painful disorder characterized by the presence of a well-circumscribed ulcer in the distal anal canal with persistent symptoms for more than 2 months (McCallion and Gardiner 2001). Chronic anal fissure results from contraction of the internal anal sphincter and is consistently associated with pain from sphincter spasm. Fissures typically present with small amounts of bright red rectal bleeding but are accompanied by constipation in only approximately 20% of patients.

9.3.2.1 Current Treatment Options

Relief of the spasm has been associated with alleviation of pain and healing of the anal fissure without recurrence. Surgical therapy, including stretch, open lateral sphincterotomy, closed lateral sphincterotomy, posterior midline sphincterotomy, and, to a lesser extent, dermal flap coverage of the fissure, has been frequently used (Nelson 2004). Sphincterotomy permanently weakens the internal sphincter and has a success rate of more than 90% but is associated with high rates of incontinence. Nonsurgical options include BoNT injection and topical agents such as nifedipine and nitroglycerin ointment to promote healing of fissures by increasing local blood flow and reducing internal sphincter pressures until the fissure heals; however, a common side effect of nitroglycerin therapy is headache.

9.3.2.2 BoNT for Chronic Anal Fissure

A number of evidence-based systematic reviews of available treatments for chronic anal fissure found improved healing with BoNT versus placebo and versus topical nitroglycerin, with fewer long-term complications than surgical treatment and avoidance of hospitalization (Brisinda et al. 1999). Clinical studies assessing the safety and efficacy of BoNT in the treatment of chronic anal fissure has reported success rates ranging from 44% to 100%. BoNT showed greater efficacy than either placebo or nitroglycerin topic therapy. No adverse effects were noted in BoNT-treated patients compared with those treated with nitroglycerin (Brisinda et al. 1999).

Long-term studies with BoNT have found successful outcomes up to 42 months, although some patients require repeat injections (Arroyo et al. 2005). De Nardi et al. (2006) compared two nonsurgical treatments for chronic anal fissure in 30 patients treated with either 0.2% nitroglycerin ointment three times daily for 8 weeks or two 10 U onabotulinumtoxinA injections and evaluated over a 3-year follow-up time frame (De Nardi et al. 2006). Both groups showed improvement at all visits, with a slightly higher percentage of patients in the nitroglycerin group showing improvement at all visits. The healing rate at 3 years was 40% in the nitroglycerin group and 33% in the BoNT group. There were no adverse events observed in the BoNT group; three patients in the nitroglycerin group reported mild headache but did not discontinue treatment. The authors concluded that although surgical sphincterotomy remains the most effective treatment for chronic anal fissure, some patients may prefer nonsurgical treatments, and particularly in patients at risk for fecal incontinence. Nitroglycerine ointment and BoNT therapy may be considered initial nonsurgical treatments of chronic anal fissure.

9.3.3 Emerging Gastrointestinal Uses of BoNT Therapy

The results of several small, open-label trials suggest that BoNT may improve symptoms of gastroparesis (Bromer et al. 2005), perhaps because injection of BoNT into the pyloric sphincter results in decreased pyloric resistance. BoNT also may have utility in gastroesophageal reflux-related noncardiac chest pain (Wong and

Fass 2004), obstructive constipation (Maria et al. 2001), and some work has suggested possible application in obese patients, with the rationale that injection of botulinum toxin in the antrum of the stomach could induce delayed gastric emptying and satiety (Albani et al. 2005).

9.4 BoNT for Hyperhidrosis

Hyperhidrosis, an idiopathic disorder affecting approximately 1% of the population, is characterized by spontaneous excessive sweating beyond that required to return body temperature to normal. The disorder is thought to be caused by overactivity of the sweat glands in the affected area in response to metabolic, environmental, neurologic, or gustatory stimuli and may be exacerbated under conditions of stress and anxiety (Lowe et al. 2004). Primary (essential or idiopathic) hyperhidrosis is focal, typically affecting the axilla, palms, soles of the feet, or face. Primary focal hyperhidrosis, which usually appears in the second or third decade of life, is often associated with a family history of the disorder. Secondary or generalized hyperhidrosis affects the entire body surface and is usually caused by underlying disease (Naumann and Jost 2004).

9.4.1 Therapeutic Approaches for Hyperhidrosis

Treatments of hyperhidrosis include systemic and topical pharmacologic agents and surgery (Eisenach et al. 2005). Topical treatments include aluminum salts, which, although often effective, are short acting and can irritate skin. Systemic medications (anticholinergics, beta blockers) have limited efficacy and substantial side effects. Surgical treatment of axillary or palmar hyperhidrosis consists of excision of the sweat glands, subcutaneous curettage and liposuction, or sympathectomy, usually performed endoscopically. Excisional surgery can be complicated by infection, bleeding, and significant scarring. Palmar hyperhidrosis may be treated topically, with iontophoresis, or by endoscopic transthoracic sympathectomy. Subcutaneous curettage and liposuction offers permanent efficacy and has fewer side effects and less scarring than excisional procedures.

9.4.2 The Role of BoNT in Hyperhidrosis Treatment

The recognized ability of BoNT to block cholinergic transmission at the neuromuscular junction and the release of acetylcholine from cholinergic postganglionic sympathetic neurons has revolutionized the treatment of autonomic hypersecretory disorders (Cohen and Solish 2003). Since eccrine sweat glands are innervated by sympathetic nerve fibers and stimulated via cholinergic neurotransmission, BoNT blockade of cholinergic autonomic nerve endings that innervate the eccrine sweat glands reduces hypersecretion of sweat.

> **Expert Opinions: Sweat Glands vs. Prostate**
> Prof. Dr. Markus Naumann
> Head of the Department of Neurology and Clinical Neurophysiology
> Klinikum Augsburg
> Stenglinstrasse 7
> 86156 Augsburg
> Germany
>
> Apart from generalized weakness, autonomic symptoms are frequent signs of the clinical spectrum of botulism due to sympathetic and parasympathetic cholinergic chemodenervation by botulinum toxin. The German physician to whose merit is the first accurate and detailed description of the clinical symptoms of food botulism – mentioned in his publications a number of autonomic disorders arising from botulism. He described in his monograph, for example, that the tear fluid disappears, no saliva is secreted, and no ear wax appears in the auditory canal. Interestingly, he also observed changes in the urogenital system such as the loss of sperm secretion and the decrease of testicles. Based on his observations, he discussed the possibility of using the toxin as a remedy for diseases associated with autonomic hyperfunction. Around 20 years ago his vision became reality by modern medicine with the first reports on successful treatment of excessive focal sweat secretion with botulinum toxin.
>
> Other indications such as drooling, Frey's syndrome or hyperlacrimation soon followed proving the principle that the local blockade of cholinergic transmission in tissues with autonomic innervation may be an excellent treatment option. It was only a consequent step to add benign prostate hyperplasia (BPH) to the spectrum of possible indications for botulinum toxin use in non-motor disorders. The first treatment results in this novel indication are very encouraging and share a number of characteristics that have previously been observed in botulinum toxin treatment of hypersecretory disorders of the sweat and salivary glands. However, many questions remain to be answered: why is the duration of botulinum toxin action in the autonomic nervous system much longer than in somatomotor nerves, frequently exceeding 6 months. Which neurotransmitters other than acetylcholine are involved in all these autonomic disorders potentially being blocked by botulinum toxin. What is the long-term effect of botulinum toxin on smooth muscle function and structure. A challenge for future research!

9.4.3 Clinical Studies of BoNT: Axillary Hyperhidrosis

OnabotulinumtoxinA was approved by the FDA in 2004 for the treatment of primary axillary hyperhidrosis. Clinical efficacy and safety was demonstrated in large-scale clinical trials. In one 16-week study, 320 patients with bilateral primary axillary hyperhidrosis were treated with 50 U onabotulinumtoxinA per axilla or placebo delivered by 10–15 intradermal injections evenly distributed within the hyperhidrotic area

(Naumann and Lowe 2001). Compared with placebo, onabotulinumtoxinA reduced sweating at all time points after administration, with response documented in 95% of BoNT recipients versus 32% of placebo-treated subjects at 1 week, 94% versus 36% at 4 weeks, and 82% versus 21% at 16 weeks. At the end of the study, 77% of BoNT patients were persistent responders compared with 18% of placebo patients.

In another large, randomized, double-blind, placebo-controlled trial, 145 patients whose rate of sweat production exceeded 50 mg/min and had hyperhidrosis unresponsive to topical treatment were injected with abobotulinumtoxinA 200 U in one axilla and placebo in the other (Heckmann et al. 2001). Two weeks later, axilla originally receiving placebo were injected with 100 U abobotulinumtoxinA. Two weeks after the initial injections, mean rates of sweat production in the abobotulinumtoxinA-treated axilla dropped from 165 to 24 mg/min compared with 174–144 mg/min in placebo axilla. Two weeks after abobotulinumtoxinA injection into axilla originally treated with placebo, the rate was 32 mg/min. At 26 weeks, sweat production rates remained lower than baseline in all BoNT-treated axilla. RimabotulinumtoxinB has also been shown to be effective in treating axillary hyperhidrosis (Dressler et al. 2002).

9.4.4 Clinical Studies of BoNT: Palmar Hyperhidrosis

Studies of BoNT in palmar hyperhidrosis have been more limited and less consistent than those in axillary hyperhidrosis because of the difficulty in maintaining a consistent injection technique and a wider range of individual susceptibility to treatment. Moreover, palmar injections are frequently painful and may require use of a nerve block of the median and ulnar nerves (Lowe et al. 2004).

In a prospective, single-blind, parallel-group trial in 24 patients with severe palmar hyperhidrosis, onabotulinumtoxinA 50 or 100 U was injected intradermally in 20 sites in each palm (Saadia et al. 2001). In the first month, there was a significant decrease in sweating that was still evident after 6 months in two thirds of patients. Although no effect on grip strength was noted, finger pinch strength decreased 2 weeks after the injection. In a double-blind, randomized, placebo-controlled trial, in which 19 patients received placebo injections in one hand and onabotulinumtoxinA in the other (Lowe et al. 2002), there was a steady decline in sweat production during 28 days following treatment and 100% of patients assessed for patient satisfaction rated treatment as successful. No concomitant decrease in grip strength or finger dexterity was reported. There were no serious adverse events.

9.4.5 BoNT for Drooling

Sialorrhea or drooling commonly affects neurologically impaired patients, including those with cerebral palsy, amyotrophic lateral sclerosis, and Parkinson's disease. BoNT can reduce saliva production by blocking acetylcholine release at the neurosecretory junction of the salivary glands (Giess et al. 2000).

A controlled, open-label, clinical trial compared two episodes of treatment of drooling in children with cerebral palsy. The first episode utilized scopolamine applied as a patch behind the ear and the second utilized submandibular BoNT injections (scopolamine was applied before BoNT because the washout period of scopolamine is known) (Jongerius et al. 2004). An assessment was scheduled on the 10th day after the initial scopolamine treatment, with the fourth patch in situ being applied no longer than 48 h before. After a washout period of 2–4 weeks, BoNT was injected. BoNT was associated with an approximately 50% response rate and a significant reduction in drooling, with maximal effect 2–8 weeks after injection. BoNT injections were associated with fewer and less serious side effects than applications of scopolamine.

9.5 Conclusions

We do not anticipate urogynecologists and urologists from around the world to be doing much botulinum toxin injection into the gastrointestinal tract, sweat glands, or facial muscles. We do anticipate that a high level understanding of why botulinum toxin has been so successfully utilized in these other medical specialties support its rationale as a treatment for the urinary bladder, prostate, and pelvic floor pain trigger points.

References

Albani G, Petroni ML, Mauro A, Liuzzi A, Lezzi G, Verti B, Marzullo P, Cattani L (2005) Safety and efficacy of therapy with botulinum toxin in obesity: a pilot study. J Gastroenterol 40(8):833–835

Aoki KR (2003) Evidence for antinociceptive activity of botulinum toxin type A in pain management. Headache 43(Suppl 1):S9–S15

Arroyo A, Perez F, Serrano P, Candela F, Calpena R (2005) Long-term results of botulinum toxin for the treatment of chronic anal fissure: prospective clinical and manometric study. Int J Colorectal Dis 20(3):267–271

Blumenfeld A (2003) Expert advice on treating migraine with botulinum toxin. Pract Neurol 2:34–41

Blumenfeld AM, Binder W, Silberstein SD, Blitzer A (2003) Procedures for administering botulinum toxin type A for migraine and tension-type headache. Headache 43(8):884–891

Brisinda G, Maria G, Bentivoglio AR, Cassetta E, Gui D, Albanese A (1999) A comparison of injections of botulinum toxin and topical nitroglycerin ointment for the treatment of chronic anal fissure. N Engl J Med 341(2):65–69

Bromer MQ, Friedenberg F, Miller LS, Fisher RS, Swartz K, Parkman HP (2005) Endoscopic pyloric injection of botulinum toxin A for the treatment of refractory gastroparesis. Gastrointest Endosc 61(7):833–839

Cohen JL, Solish N (2003) Treatment of hyperhidrosis with botulinum toxin. Facial Plast Surg Clin North Am 11(4):493–502

Cuilliere C, Ducrotte P, Zerbib F, Metman EH, de Looze D, Guillemot F, Hudziak H, Lamouliatte H, Grimaud JC, Ropert A, Dapoigny M, Bost R, Lemann M, Bigard MA, Denis P, Auget JL, Galmiche JP, Bruley des Varannes S (1997) Achalasia: outcome of patients treated with intrasphincteric injection of botulinum toxin. Gut 41(1):87–92

De Andres J, Cerda-Olmedo G, Valia JC, Monsalve V, Lopez A, Minguez A (2003) Use of botulinum toxin in the treatment of chronic myofascial pain. Clin J Pain 19(4):269–275

De Nardi P, Ortolano E, Radaelli G, Staudacher C (2006) Comparison of glycerine trinitrate and botulinum toxin-a for the treatment of chronic anal fissure: long-term results. Dis Colon Rectum 49(4):427–432

Difazio M, Jabbari B (2002) A focused review of the use of botulinum toxins for low back pain. Clin J Pain 18(6 Suppl):S155–S162

Dressler D, Adib Saberi F, Benecke R (2002) Botulinum toxin type B for treatment of axillar hyperhidrosis. J Neurol 249(12):1729–1732

Eisenach JH, Atkinson JL, Fealey RD (2005) Hyperhidrosis: evolving therapies for a well-established phenomenon. Mayo Clin Proc 80(5):657–666

Evers S, Vollmer-Haase J, Schwaag S, Rahmann A, Husstedt IW, Frese A (2004) Botulinum toxin A in the prophylactic treatment of migraine – a randomized, double-blind, placebo-controlled study. Cephalalgia 24(10):838–843

Ferrante FM, Bearn L, Rothrock R, King L (2005) Evidence against trigger point injection technique for the treatment of cervicothoracic myofascial pain with botulinum toxin type A. Anesthesiology 103(2):377–383

Foster L, Clapp L, Erickson M, Jabbari B (2001) Botulinum toxin A and chronic low back pain: a randomized, double-blind study. Neurology 56(10):1290–1293

Friedenberg F, Gollamudi S, Parkman HP (2004) The use of botulinum toxin for the treatment of gastrointestinal motility disorders. Dig Dis Sci 49(2):165–175

Garofalo JH, Pofahl WE (2002) Achalasia: a brief review of treatment options and efficacy. Curr Surg 59(6):549–553

Giess R, Naumann M, Werner E, Riemann R, Beck M, Puls I, Reiners C, Toyka KV (2000) Injections of botulinum toxin A into the salivary glands improve sialorrhoea in amyotrophic lateral sclerosis. J Neurol Neurosurg Psychiatry 69(1):121–123

Han SC, Harrison P (1997) Myofascial pain syndrome and trigger-point management. Reg Anesth 22(1):89–101

Heckmann M, Ceballos-Baumann AO, Plewig G (2001) Botulinum toxin A for axillary hyperhidrosis (excessive sweating). N Engl J Med 344(7):488–493

Jongerius PH, Rotteveel JJ, van Limbeek J, Gabreels FJ, van Hulst K, van den Hoogen FJ (2004) Botulinum toxin effect on salivary flow rate in children with cerebral palsy. Neurology 63(8):1371–1375

Kaufman JA, Oelschlager BK (2005) Treatment of Achalasia. Curr Treat Options Gastroenterol 8(1):59–69

Lang AM (2004) Botulinum toxin type B in piriformis syndrome. Am J Phys Med Rehabil 83(3):198–202

Lipton RB, Scher AI, Kolodner K, Liberman J, Steiner TJ, Stewart WF (2002) Migraine in the United States: epidemiology and patterns of health care use. Neurology 58(6):885–894

Lipton RB, Stewart WF, Diamond S, Diamond ML, Reed M (2001) Prevalence and burden of migraine in the United States: data from the American Migraine Study II. Headache 41(7):646–657

Lowe N, Campanati A, Bodokh I, Cliff S, Jaen P, Kreyden O, Naumann M, Offidani A, Vadoud J, Hamm H (2004) The place of botulinum toxin type A in the treatment of focal hyperhidrosis. Br J Dermatol 151(6):1115–1122

Lowe NJ, Yamauchi PS, Lask GP, Patnaik R, Iyer S (2002) Efficacy and safety of botulinum toxin type a in the treatment of palmar hyperhidrosis: a double-blind, randomized, placebo-controlled study. Dermatol Surg 28(9):822–827

Maria G, Brisinda G, Bentivoglio AR, Albanese A, Sganga G, Castagneto M (2001) Anterior rectocele due to obstructed defecation relieved by botulinum toxin. Surgery 129(5):524–529

McCallion K, Gardiner KR (2001) Progress in the understanding and treatment of chronic anal fissure. Postgrad Med J 77(914):753–758

Moskowitz MA (1993) Neurogenic inflammation in the pathophysiology and treatment of migraine. Neurology 43(6 Suppl 3):S16–S20

Naumann M, Jost W (2004) Botulinum toxin treatment of secretory disorders. Mov Disord 19(Suppl 8):S137–S141

Naumann M, Lowe NJ (2001) Botulinum toxin type A in treatment of bilateral primary axillary hyperhidrosis: randomised, parallel group, double blind, placebo controlled trial. BMJ 323(7313):596–599

Nelson R (2004) A systematic review of medical therapy for anal fissure. Dis Colon Rectum 47(4):422–431

Opida C (2002) Evaluation of Myobloc (botulinum toxin type B) in patients with post-whiplash headaches. Pain Med 3:178–179

Pasricha PJ, Ravich WJ, Hendrix TR, Sostre S, Jones B, Kalloo AN (1995) Intrasphincteric botulinum toxin for the treatment of achalasia. N Engl J Med 332(12):774–778

Porta M (2000) A comparative trial of botulinum toxin type A and methylprednisolone for the treatment of myofascial pain syndrome and pain from chronic muscle spasm. Pain 85(1–2):101–105

Ramadan NM (2003) The link between glutamate and migraine. CNS Spectr 8(6):446–449

Saadia D, Voustianiouk A, Wang AK, Kaufmann H (2001) Botulinum toxin type A in primary palmar hyperhidrosis: randomized, single-blind, two-dose study. Neurology 57(11):2095–2099

Silberstein S, Mathew N, Saper J, Jenkins S (2000) Botulinum toxin type A as a migraine preventive treatment. For the BOTOX Migraine Clinical Research Group. Headache 40(6):445–450

Smith CP, Somogyi GT, Chancellor MB (2002a) Botulinum toxin treatment of urethral and bladder dysfunction. Int Braz J Urol 28(6):545–552

Smith CP, Somogyi GT, Chancellor MB (2002b) Emerging role of botulinum toxin in the treatment of neurogenic and non-neurogenic voiding dysfunction. Curr Urol Rep 3(5):382–387

Troost BT (2004) Botulinum toxin type A (Botox) in the treatment of migraine and other headaches. Expert Rev Neurother 4(1):27–31

Wong WM, Fass R (2004) Noncardiac chest pain. Curr Treat Options Gastroenterol 7(4):273–278

Health Economics of Botulinum Toxin Application

10.1 Introduction

It may be a surprise to many that with over 3 billion dollars in annual sales of antimuscarinic drugs globally, fewer than 30% of patients remain on antimuscarinic therapy 1 year after initiating therapy for overactive bladder (OAB). Suboptimal efficacy and anticholinergic side effects challenge adherence to antimuscarinic drugs (Haab and Castro-Diaz 2005).

Procedures that can be considered for antimuscarinic refractory patients include sacral neuromodulation, injection of botulinum toxin (BoNT) and augmentation cystoplasty. Sacral neuromodulation and BoNT are less invasive with a diminished risk profile versus open bladder surgeries such as augmentation cystoplasty (Greenwell et al. 2001).

With OAB related costs estimated at over $12 billion US dollars (Hu et al. 2003), healthcare decision makers are becoming interested in evaluating the cost of sacral neuromodulation, BoNT and augmentation cystoplasty for overactive bladder patients refractory to antimuscarinic therapy. It is only recently that the potential health economic impact of bladder BoNT has been researched and we will look at some of the recent data.

10.2 Sacral Nerve Neuromodulation

The use of sacral nerve neuromodulation is based on the premise that electrical stimulation of the sacral nerves can modulate neural reflexes that influence bladder and pelvic floor behavior. The approved indications for sacral nerve neuromodulation include refractory OAB, urinary retention, and bowel dysfunction in a number of developed countries.

For patients with OAB, the device is tested using an external stimulator for a trial period of days to weeks. The external stimulator is considered to be successful when the symptoms improve by at least 50%; if this device is successful, a permanent stimulator is implanted, which can later be removed if necessary.

10.2.1 Clinical Results with Sacral Nerve Neuromodulation

A systematic review, which included data from patients with 1,827 implants, reported a >50% improvement in urgency urinary incontinence in over two third of patients (Brazzelli et al. 2006). Incontinence episodes, leakage severity, voiding frequency, and pad use were significantly lower after implantation, and benefits were reported to persist for up to 3–5 years.

Adverse effects most commonly reported include pain at the lead or implant site, new pain such as leg pain and infection of devices. Reoperation rate was reported to be 33%. The full mechanism of action of sacral nerve neuromodulation remains incompletely understood.

10.3 Comparative Cost Analysis

How does bladder botulinum toxin injection stack up versus established procedures of augmentation cystoplasty and sacral neuromodulation? One of the earlier BoNT analyses was by Kalsi et al. (2006) who reported that BoNT therapy for neurogenic or idiopathic detrusor overactivity costs British Pounds £826 per patient, with a cost-effectiveness ratio of £617 per patient-year with ≥25% clinical improvement.

Watanabe et al. (2010) recently published a cost analysis of resource use for sacral neuromodulation, BoNT and augmentation cystoplasty from a United States payer perspective. Resource use included inpatient services, outpatient services, pharmaceuticals, and physician payments. Resource use was converted to costs using standardized fee schedules to generate national average estimates. The approach to costing was based on literature review of other OAB cost research performed and review of billing and guidance literature.

Costs in 2007 US dollars were calculated and sensitivity analyses were performed to evaluate assumptions and uncertainty of results based on plausible variation in estimates of key cost drivers. Injection of BoNT is generally performed as a 1-h procedure in a physician's office. Hence, costing was limited to physician costs via procedure codes and BoNT procurement cost using average selling price schedules. Procedure codes for augmentation cystoplasty were determined based on descriptions from the literature. For calculations of sacral neuromodulation costs beyond year 1, a 33% probability of revision and average number of two reprograms per year were used. BoNT costs beyond 1 year were calculated by assuming continued injection of BoNT at 6 month intervals.

10.3.1 Results

Sacral neuromodulation initial procedure costs were related to the test stimulation, implantation of the pulse generator, insertion of electrodes, and programming. The initial surgical center cost included payments to the facility for the procedures and payment for the implanted medical device. Injection of BoNT initial procedure

10.3 Comparative Cost Analysis

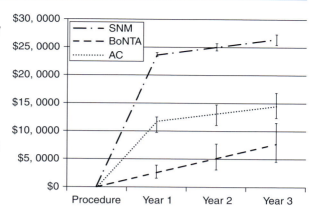

Fig. 10.1 Estimated cumulative cost curve in 2007 US dollars. Bands delineate minimum and maximum costs based on sensitivity analyses. *SNM* sacral nerve neuromodulation, *BoNTA* botulinum toxin-A, *AC* augmentation cystoplasty (Watanabe et al. 2010. Copyright 2010 Elsevier Inc.)

Table 10.1 Initial treatment cost of the three treatment modalities in 2007 US dollars

Treatment	Drug costs	Procedure costs	Facility costs	Total costs
Sacral nerve neuromodulation	N.A[a]	$2,289	$19,937	$22,226
OnabotulinumtoxinA	$1,052	$261	N/A[b]	$1,313
Augmentation cystoplasty	N.A[a]	$1,072	$9,180	$10,252

Modified from Watanabe et al. 2010
[a]Drug and device costs included in facility costs
[b]Office procedure with no facility costs

costs were related to cystoscopy and injection using BoNT as an office-based procedure with no affiliated surgical center payment. Augmentation cystoplasty initial procedure and surgical center costs were delineated by specified codes and assumptions of a 34% complication rate.

The initial treatment cost was US Dollars $22,226; $1,313; and $10,252 for sacral neuromodulation, injection of BoNT, and augmentation cystoplasty, respectively. Three years after initiating treatment, the cumulative cost was $26,269; $7,651; and $14,337, respectively (Fig. 10.1 and Table 10.1).

Estimated cumulative cost at the end of year 3 for sacral neuromodulation exceeded the cost of injection of BoNT by $18,718. Estimated cumulative cost at the end of year 3 for sacral neuromodulation exceeded the cost of augmentation cystoplasty by $12,032. There are little long-term studies with these interventions.

Limitations of this study include the fact that costs were estimated using literature sources for duration of continued effect and adverse effect probabilities. The lack of robust long-term efficacy and safety studies for these procedures introduces uncertainty in these cost estimates. Without regulatory approved dosing, BoNT costs are projected based on literature-based practice patterns.

10.4 Other Recent Reports

Health economics of BoNT is a new topic and it is only recently that interesting new reports are being presented.

10.4.1 BoNT Versus Anticholinergics

Wu et al., (2009) from Duke University in the United States assessed the cost-effectiveness of BoNT injection compared to anticholinergic medications for the treatment of idiopathic urgency incontinence. They used a Markov decision analysis model to compare the costs in 2008 U.S. dollars and effectiveness in quality adjusted life-years.

The analysis was conducted with a 2-year time frame using 3-month cycles. The primary outcome was the incremental cost-effectiveness ratio, defined as the difference from BoNT minus anticholinergic cost divided by the difference in BoNT minus anticholinergic quality adjusted life-years.

Wu and associates noted that while BoNT was more expensive (US dollars $4,392 vs. $2,563) it was also more effective (1.63 vs. 1.50 quality adjusted life-years) compared to anticholinergics. The calculated incremental cost-effectiveness ratio was $14,377 per quality adjusted life-year. Most cost outcome research considers a new treatment cost-effective, when the incremental cost-effectiveness ratio is less than $50,000 per quality adjusted life-year. It should be noted that anticholinergics become cost-effective if patients are compliant with medications, or if the BoNT procedure costs increase substantially.

10.4.2 BoNT Versus Augmentation Cystoplasty

Padmanabhan and associates (2010) from Vanderbilt University in the United States compared bladder BoNT with augmentation cystoplasty with estimation of the average initial treatment costs and cumulative 5 year costs. A survey of literature provided the percentages of outcomes and complications while procedure fee were taken from databases reported in 2008–2009 US dollars.

It estimated the initial treatment costs were US dollars $25,042 for augmentation cystoplasty and $2,947 BoNT-A. Long-term costs were calculated based on success, failure, and complications of BoNT-A and augmentation cystoplasty. The average cumulative 5 year cost by intervention was $33,272 for augmentation cystoplasty and $28,065 for bi-annual BoNT injections. This study demonstrated BoNT as the more cost effective choice over a 5-year period in the treatment of neurogenic bladder patients. If the complications rate of augmentation cystoplasty falls below 14%, surgery may be more advantageous.

10.4.3 Different Brands of Botulinum Toxin

This is one of the first cost comparisons between two types of BoNT-A: abobotulinumtoxinA, (Ipsen Ltd, Slough, UK) and onabotulinumtoxinA (Allergan Inc., Irvine, USA), in the treatment of patients with idiopathic detrusor overactivity. Robinson and associates (2010a, b) from Preston Hospital, United Kingdom compared the cost and benefit of treatment with either 500 U abobotulinumtoxinA or 200 U onabotulinumtoxinA.

The number of patients reviewed was not stated but the authors reported there were no identifiable subjective or objective outcome differences between groups. However, there was a cost saving of British pound £119.40 using abobotulinumtoxinA compared to onabotulinumtoxinA at the specific doses used in this study.

10.4.4 BoNT Cost to the French Health Care System

Campbell and associates (2010) estimated the costs and outcomes of onabotulinumtoxinA compared to standard of care for the treatment of urinary incontinence in spinal cord injury patients using the French payer perspective. A Markov model was used to evaluate two different treatment strategies in patients who failed oral antimuscarinics. In the standard-of-care arm, patients were assumed to have no further pharmacologic treatment with only a subgroup of patients undergoing augmentation cystoplasty. In the onabotulinumtoxinA arm, all patients were assumed to have been treated with 300 U of onabotulinumtoxinA.

OnabotulinumtoxinA non-responders were assumed to have no further pharmacologic treatment, but a subgroup of them received augmentation cystoplasty. A 50% reduction in incontinence episodes was considered treatment success, and a 7.5 month onabotulinumtoxinA retreatment time interval was used as a successful treatment outcome. Model outputs included health care resource utilization, quality-adjusted survival year, payer costs, and incremental cost-effectiveness ratio (ICER).

The onabotulinumtoxinA treatment strategy as compared to standard of care resulted in a 10 year incremental cost of Euro €11,048, 0.43 quality-adjusted survival gained, and a cost-effectiveness ratio of €25,580/quality-adjusted survival year. The estimated additional cost per onabotulinumtoxinA treated patient-year to the French payer was €1,105. The financial impact of adding onabotulinumtoxinA treatment in this population for the French payer was €0.14 per French person-year.

At less than €30,000/quality-adjusted survival year, onabotulinumtoxinA may be considered good value from the French payer's perspective. Due to the relatively small population of eligible patients, the cost impact would be expected to be small on the overall healthcare budget.

10.4.5 BoNT Versus New Modalities

Robinson and associates from the Kings College Hospital, London, United Kingdom, (2010a, b) studied refractory OAB patients with cost utility analysis of BoNT versus the new technique of percutaneous tibial nerve stimulation. A decision analytic Markov model was developed to compare the cost-utility of percutaneous tibial nerve stimulation and BoNT with 2 year follow-up period and costing using England's National Health Service perspective in patients with refractory idiopathic OAB.

The annual equivalent cost of the device was calculated assuming a life span of 5 years. A cost per use of the device was then estimated under the assumption that the equipment would be used five times per week. Percutaneous tibial stimulation involved 12 weekly visits and subsequent maintenance therapy of one session per month. For BoNT, drug costs were estimated using the British National Formulary for onabotulinumtoxinA 200 U. It was assumed that patients would have repeat treatments every 8 months in the out-patient setting and clean intermittent catheterization rates were assumed to be 20% for an interval of 4 months. It was assumed that patients would drop out following unsuccessful treatment.

In line with standard NICE (National Institute of Health and Clinical Excellence) methodology, costs and effects in year 2 were discounted at 3.5%. It was assumed that a patient would have a 0.02 increase in health state utility as a result of improvement and a 0.05 gain from cure. The incremental cost effectiveness ratio of each treatment was calculated relative to the next most effective treatment or 'do nothing'. Sensitivity analysis was undertaken to explore the impact of assumptions about the gains in health state utility from successful treatment.

In the best case analysis comparison, percutaneous tibial nerve stimulation therapy was found to be cheaper than botulinum toxin (British Pound £1,700.00 and £4,067.00 respectively; difference − £2,367.00). However, neither would be considered cost-effective using the advisory willingness to pay the threshold often adopted in NICE guidance (£20,000–£30,000 per quality-adjusted survival year).

This study suggests that percutaneous tibial nerve stimulation therapy may be cheaper than treatment with BoNT in women with refractory idiopathic OAB. This finding is highly sensitive to the assumptions about the extent to which cure and improvement would improve health related quality of life. If a relatively low improvement in health state utility is assumed, neither treatment would appear to be cost effective.

10.5 Conclusion

With OAB related costs estimated at over $12 billion just in the United States, the health economic impact of each treatment modality must also be factored when considering the choice of therapy. Future studies should prospectively address cost-benefit-risk of treatment options for neurogenic and nonneurogenic overactive bladder so that clinicians and their patients can make informed, and well-educated choices.

References

Brazzelli M, Murray A, Fraser C (2006) Efficacy and safety of sacral nerve stimulation for urinary urge incontinence: a systematic review. J Urol 175:835–841

Campbell J, Velard M, Denys P, Chartier-Kastler E, Kowalski J, Sullivan S (2010) Cost-effectiveness and financial impact of onabotulinumtoxinA treatment for urinary incontinence due to neurogenic detrusor overactivity in spinal cord injury patients within the French healthcare system. ICS. Abstract 358

Greenwell TJ, Venn SN, Mundy AR (2001) Augmentation cystoplasty. BJU Int 88:511–525

Haab H, Castro-Diaz D (2005) Persistence with antimuscarinic therapy in patients with overactive bladder. Int J Clin Pract 59:931–937

Hu T, Wagner TH, Benkover JD (2003) Estimated costs of overactive bladder in the United States. Urology 61:1123–1128, 2003

Kalsi V, Popat RB, Apostolidis A, Kavia R, Odeyemi IA, Dakin HA, Warner J, Elneil S, Fowler CJ, Dasgupta P (2006) Cost-consequence analysis evaluating the use of botulinum neurotoxin-A in patients with detrusor overactivity based on clinical outcomes observed at a single UK centre. Eur Urol 49:519–527

Padmanabhan P, Scarpero H, Milam D, Dmochowski R, Penson D. 5 year cost analysis of intra-detrusor injection of botulinum toxin type A and augmentation cystoplasty for refractory neurogenic detrusor overactivity. ICS. 2010. Abstract 530

Robinson R, Moore K, Haq A (2010a) Dysport® versus Botox® in the treatment of idiopathic detrusor overactivity. A financial and outcome evaluation. ICS. Abstract 354

Robinson D, Jacklin P, Cardozo L (2010b) What's needling us about the management of refractory overactive bladder? An economic analysis of the use of percutaneous tibial nerve stimulation and botulinum toxin. ICS. Abstract 180

Watanabe JH, Campbell JD, Ravelo A, Chancellor MB, Kowalski J, Sullivan S (2010) Cost analysis of interventions for antimuscarinic refractory patients with overactive bladder. Urology 76:835–840

Wu JM, Siddiqui NY, Amundsen CL, Myers ER, Havrilesky LJ, Visco AG (2009) Cost-effectiveness of botulinum toxin a versus anticholinergic medications for idiopathic urge incontinence. J Urol 181:2181–2186

Perspectives from Around the World: Panorama of Where We Are and Where We Are Going

11.1 Australia: Jeffrey Thavaseelan

In Australia it is estimated that within the next 10 years, health care costs related to the management of urinary incontinence will be in the order of 1.2 billion dollars annually. The prevalence of urinary incontinence in Australia is estimated at between 34% and 45% in women and between 4% and 15% in men depending on the criteria used and subpopulations studied.

The overactive bladder, both neurogenic and non-neurogenic, understandably contributes to the prevalence of urinary incontinence. In the past, those who failed medical therapy had little choice but to suffer in silence or to commit to major operative intervention. In the neurogenic group, especially those with spinal cord injury, we perform an enterocystoplasty which is still an acceptable option. However, in the non-neurogenic population such major surgery is not seen favorably by the patient. Other surgical procedures such as trigonal isolation and phenol injections have not endured the test of time.

The introduction of botulinum toxin has revolutionized the management of the overactive bladder in Australia. Although it has been trialed in a few specialized centers since 2002, it was not until 2006 that the use of Botulinum toxin became popular among urologists and urogynecologists. In 2005, under the auspices of the Urological Society of Australia and New Zealand, we conducted the first Australian Workshop on this subject.

Botulinum toxin is now an accepted part of the treatment algorithm for patients with neurogenic overactivity who have failed medical therapy with anticholinergic medication. As a consequence, many patients have avoided progression to an enterocystoplasty. In the non-neurogenic group however, treatment with botulinum toxin is less widespread, though I expect this to change with time and experience. A major limiting factor has been the concern regarding urinary retention, which should abate as further trials are published and doses are more established. In addition, the recent approval in Australia of the use of sacral neuromodulation has created competition in an area that not so long ago was devoid of any minimally invasive options.

Other areas for which botulinum toxin has been used in Australia include detrusor sphincter dyssynergia, chronic bladder pain, and pediatric urology, specifically in patients with congenital spinal pathology. A major issue that we are faced with in Australia is cost. At present, botulinum toxin is not Therapeutic Goods Administration approved for urological indications and is thus not eligible for the government rebate. Despite this, with increased awareness by health authorities and pressure from patients, several specialized government hospitals have chosen to fund the use of botulinum toxin in specific subgroups of patients. In the private hospital setting, the costs are either borne by the patient or in some cases by the health insurance company.

Botulinum toxin has definitely become part of the urologist's armamentarium in Australia. However its endurance is dependent on bureaucratic decisions and the recognition that this important treatment option will save health care costs in the long term.

Dr. Jeffrey Thavaseelan, M.B.B.S., F.R.A.C.S.
Head of Neurourology and Urodynamics Unit
Royal Perth Rehabilitation Hospital
Perth, Western Australia
Consultant Urologist
UrologyWest
Suite 52 SJOG Murdoch Medical Centre

11.2 Belgium: Dirk De Ridder

OnabotulinumtoxinA is being used in Belgium since 1999, a year after the first publications by Stöhrer and Schurch. Initially it was used in neurogenic bladders, especially in patients with multiple sclerosis. Gradually the indications expanded from patients practicing intermittent catheterization, with urine leakage in between catheterizations, to patients with indwelling catheters and persistent leakage to patients who did not catheterize but suffered from refractory detrusor overactivity.

Despite the fact that no reimbursement was offered for this treatment the acceptance by the patients was high because of the excellent effects of this treatment. The treatments were done as outpatient procedures under local anesthesia.

After a few years, idiopathic OAB was developed as a new indication. We usually used 100 U onabotulinumtoxinA as standard dose for this indication. This dose proved to an acceptable benefit/risk ratio (especially retention and intermittent catheterization), while the cost was still acceptable for most patients.

New indications a under investigation include chronic pelvic pain, and female dyspareunia due to pelvic floor spasticity.

In summary this drug has lead to an impressive improvement in the management of overactive bladder in neurological disease and in idiopathic OAB. A knowledge progresses, new indications will arise and it is a privilege to be a part of these evolutions.

Professor Dr. Dirk De Ridder
kliniekhoofd urologie UZ Leuven
hoofdgeneesheer Nationaal MS Centrum
UZ Leuven | campus Gasthuisberg | Herestraat 49 | B – 3000 Leuven |

11.3 Canada: Sender Herschorn

In 2008, total healthcare expenditures in Canada were $171.8 billion (CAD) (CIHI 2010) and were expected to rise to $182.1 billion in 2009 and $191.6 billion in 2010. In 1997 dollars the rate of increase from $40 billion in 1975 to $131 billion in 2008 was 227.5% and paralleled the yearly rate of inflation. In 2008 total health expenditure was 10.4% of gross domestic product. The United States was higher at 16% followed by France at 11.2%. Nine European countries were within one percentage point of Canada's spending.

The public sector share of Canada's healthcare spending has reached 70.6% of the total, reflecting the character of a publicly financed system. Spending on drugs has become the second largest category of expenditures after hospitals and now amounts to $31 billion or 16.3% of overall expenditures. The private sector (insurance companies and self-pay) share of drug costs is 53.5% in contrast to 29.4% for overall health spending (CIHI 2010).

The funding in Canada for overactive bladder drugs is similarly complex. Approval of a drug is through the federal Ministry of Health and each province sets its own rules for publicly funded formulary coverage. Most overactive bladder drugs are not covered in public formularies while private insurance usually covers them. This may explain why most drugs are available in this country but access to them is restricted.

The prevalence of overactive bladder symptoms has been well documented in different population-based studies in Canada. Corcos and Schick (2004) reported the overall prevalence at 18.1% (14.8% of men and 21.2% of women). Subsequently, Herschorn et al. (2008) reported the overall prevalence at 13.9% (13.1% of men and 14.7% of women). Milsom and Irwin (2007) in the EPIC study noted prevalence in Canada of approximately 10%. Overall about 2–4 million Canadian adults have overactive bladder symptoms.

The advent of botulinum toxin for neurogenic and idiopathic overactive bladder opens another avenue of therapy. Clinical trials are demonstrating efficacy and safety in anticholinergic refractory patients. Health Canada approval for its use will probably come through and private insurers will also most likely cover it. However, public formulary coverage is not guaranteed and cystoscopy is only publicly funded. The challenge will be to provide access for all patients who need it in a healthcare system where increasing costs have mandated cost constraints and prioritization of problems. Overactive bladder and incontinence have not been prioritized.

Sender Herschorn, B.Sc., M.D.C.M., F.R.C.S.C.
Head of Urodynamic Unit and Attending Urologist
Professor Division of Urology/Department of Surgery

University of Toronto
Sunnybrook Health Sciences Centre
2075 Bayview Avenue
Toronto, ON M4N 3M5
Canada

11.4 France: Emmanuel Chartier-Kastler

Ever since the presentation of Brigitte Schurch at the International Continence Society Meeting in Denver in 1999, botulinum toxin has appeared for French neurourologists as a major revolution in the treatment of spinal cord injured patients. Finally, there was available an efficient treatment for neurogenic overactive bladder that did not require invasive surgery. Over time the evaluation of botulinum toxin obtained the attention of other French and international urologists. Quickly, evaluation of botulinum toxin for idiopathic overactivity bladder was undertaken and, outside of any labeling and official conclusion about its role in this area, some urologists came to its compassionate use for non-neurogenic patients. No company owning a botulinum toxin has ever advertised or communicated on it but the urologists in France had the strong feeling that an unusual drug with unusual therapeutic abilities was now available.

Most physicians never hear such news about a new drug, whatever the effect, before phase III trials are completed and scientific communication can be built. But this case was different. Botulinum toxin, a new agent with a new route of delivery, and with an apparent unusual efficiency was enough for one specialty to open our eyes and ears.

Whatever the final indications and labeling that will emerge in France for botulinum toxin it seems to be able to fill the gap in a therapeutic area where no other marketed drug is able to help our patients. The best advertisement that could be done for French neurourology and for multidisciplinary management of patients by rehabilitation physicians and urologists are the beneficial results of this new treatment.

The confident area of functional urology is most of the time the start of new pathophysiological concepts that can also help non-neurogenic patients suffering urge incontinence. Botulinum toxin is routinely compared to the concept of self catheterization as one of the major discoveries in this field within the last 40 years. Its impact has been more than to improve quality of life of our patients', it has also promoted the diagnosis and management of urge incontinence by urologists. How a drug can help a subspecialty image!

Now as we wait for the final evaluation of its best indications and possible approval for reimbursement, we must also develop tools to control indications for usage and to prevent bad practice. A quick acceptance of this drug may kill the drug if there are any side effects that are badly managed. We must temper the idea for patients and general urologists that botulinum toxin may be indicated for all types of voiding dysfunctions, particularly in conditions that we do not understand well or

do not always cure. Nonetheless, a great future for all of us will come when the official era of botulinum toxin therapy begins in urology!
Professor Emmanuel Chartier-Kastler, M.D., Ph.D.
Pierre et Marie Curie Medical School, Paris VI
France

11.5 Germany: Tim Schneider

The use of BoNT has become more and more popular during the last years. The first steps have been made by Manfred Stöhrer in Murnau, who started to treat neurogenic bladder dysfunction in paraplegic patients. Today BoNT is used for idiopathic overactive bladder as well as for neurogenic bladder dysfunction and in some cases in patients with benign prostatic enlargement or acute urinary retention. The main problem is that reimbursement is not provided in Germany and therefore treatment using local anaesthesia on an outpatient basis is rare. Most patients are treated with general anaesthesia and have to stay several days in the hospital in order to receive coverage by the insurance companies. Treatment is performed in most clinics with rigid cystoscopes although the use of flexible instruments is also possible.

In my opinion, the use of BoNT in urological indications will increase strongly, when reimbursement is provided by the insurance companies. Nevertheless, my personal belief is that BoNT will not be able to replace anticholinergic treatment completely due to its more invasive nature of application, but it may replace it in up to 30% of the overactive bladder population. Treatment of patients with acute urinary retention or benign prostatic enlargement may not become important because most patients will end up again with urinary retention after 6–12 months. The key to a high patient satisfaction in the overactive bladder population will be a very subtle dosage regime, starting with low doses in order to avoid urinary retention, which is for sure the most bothering adverse event in this population.

Tim Schneider, M.D.
Priv.-Doz. Dr.med. Tim Schneider
PUR/R
Praxisklinik Urologie Rhein/Ruhr
Schulstraße 11
45468 Mülheim

11.6 India Sanjay Pandey

11.6.1 Early Years of BoNT in Indian Urology (2005–2007)

Botulinum toxin applications in Indian Urology scenario coincided with a surge in understanding of OAB in India when this freshly defined scenario was seriously taken as a modern day quality of life issue while its refractoriness was undergoing the test of the evolving agents as improved options of the anticholinergic world.

Neurogenic detrusor overactivity got the much needed boost with Phase 2–3 trials distributed across academic centres in the country. BoNT did create the early niche as an attempt in minimally invasive management for refractory OAB before diving into the established "invasive" augmentation options. The early years saw submucosal and intradetrusor attempts by few neurourology centres in idiopathic and neurogenic OAB as planned admissions under general anesthesia with close monitoring. The early attempts of medical colleges to establish the BoNT programme was slow and in purely refractoriness of the status.

The initial stumbling blocks were largely the personal expenses involved by patients, the slow enthusiasm of a new unlabelled molecule, lack of availability to every attempting urologist, lack of training and complete core knowledge of the subject and techniques for the same and case selection issues. More urologists in private practice used the wonder molecule to commence their programmes with anecdotal difficult cases before convincing their peers, patients, and themselves in their long term endeavours with BoNT as myself.

11.6.2 The BoNT "Wonder Years" in Indian Urology (2008–2010)

The very strong impetus of BoNT driven clinical trials in few chosen centres across the country sprouted tremendous interest in this new therapy which is gradually getting accepted as a durable, yet reversible treatment option on selected off-label indications in bladder and external sphincter at few Neurourology centres, notably at Kokilaben Dhirubhai Ambani Hospital & Research Institute in Mumbai becoming a nodal point of referrals for the planned indications backed by extensive urodynamics study and training of juniors and enthusiastic teams with workshops and symposia. One such national live webinar from Kokilaben Dhirubhai Ambani Hospital in October 2010 on OAB evoked true and ethical considerations and improved interest and referrals in the refractory states.

The recent times from 2008 onwards saw insurance companies covering the bladder indications (except interstitial cystitis and painful bladder syndromes), enthusiastic neurourology centres taking up smaller numbers, training by us at our centre and in few recent workshops, availability of the molecule by two companies as Botox (Allergan, USA) and Neuronox (Ranbaxy, India); no significant complications or resistance while the technique evolved from treating as inpatients to day-care, from rigid to flexible scopes, from general anaesthesia to local anaesthesia and from fixed needles to adjustable needle tips.

Intraprostatic injections have not found many takers at this time with patient preferences towards complete cure from BPH. The most common usage in prostate has been in the "accepted most high risk patients" under minimal anaesthesia. The largest series was communicated from Safdarjung Hospital in New Delhi in 2008 of moderate sized prostates with comparable results. BoNT has not found favour in the much awaited interstitial cystitis/painful bladder syndromes despite the epidemiological nature of the entity being commonly discussed and reported. The usage has been largely relegated to late presentations and fibrosed bladders where results have been suboptimal. There needs to be a national registry of the interstitial cystitis cases and a genuine attempt towards upliftment of the quality of life of these syndromes by BoNT as reported in conjunction with alternative therapies the world over. With Kokilaben Dhirubhai Ambani Hospital taking up detrusor sphincter dyssenergia as a manageable entity for a select group of spinal injury and multiple sclerosis patients with repeat injections over 6–9 months, Neurourology has seen upbeat interest in the rejuvenated results of detrusor sphincter dyssynergia.

11.6.3 Challenges and Drafts for Future (2011 – Beyond)

As BoNT looks forward to regulatory approval, the onus depends on this safe therapy being taken forward to improve the fate of various complex voiding syndromes as shown by half a decade of incessant improvement in patient outcomes while the silent demand escalates. Improving training to juniors would depend on national and locoregional symposiums and workshops; guidelines and mentoring would go a long way in improving acceptability amongst fellow urology colleagues. As present applications get crystallized and embodied in shape of indications, the extraordinary molecule has a safe and conceivable future that looks upbeat in India's increasing patient numbers of established and proven lower tract indications.

Dr. Sanjay Pandey
Consultant – Department of Urology
Andrology and Gender reassignment Surgery
2nd Floor, Kokilaben Dhirubhai Ambani Hospital
Four Bungalows, Andheri West
Mumbai, 400053
India

11.7   Italy: Antonella Giannantoni

Poor outcomes of treatments for overactive bladder syndrome (OAB) and detrusor overactivity have led in recent times to a search for more efficacious therapies. Among new treatment modalities, intravesical injection of botulinum toxin has shown promise in the treatment of these conditions. Since the first report on the efficacy of the botulinum neurotoxin A in the treatment of refractory neurogenic detrusor overactivity by Schurch and co-workers (2000), there have been a number of publications documenting the application of BoNT in the treatment of a wide range of voiding dysfunction. Although still waiting for approval, since 2000 BoNT treatment has been used also in Italy in the urologic field, with enormous interest from both patients and physicians involved in neurourology and, more generally, in functional urology.

To date, BoNT injections can be offered in both university and community hospitals in different regions of Italy to well informed patients affected by various conditions as neurogenic and non-neurogenic OAB. Painful bladder syndrome/

interstitial cystitis and BPH, and hundreds of patients have been treated in Italy with BoNT for these pathologies with satisfactory results. Worth of noting, Italian researchers were the first in 2003 in using BoNT in the treatment of BPH with intraprostatic injections, thus obtaining very intriguing results (Maria et al. 2003). Of interest, Italian researches have been focused on the use of the BoNT in the treatment of painful bladder syndrome/interstitial cystitis (Giannantoni et al. 2006a), with both preliminary experiences and long term studies. Also, in recent times there has been in this country the development of laboratory research to investigate the mechanisms of action of the neurotoxin into the detrusor muscle in cooperation with international groups of experts. Particularly, some of the research include the investigation of the effects of the neurotoxin on bladder neurotransmitters as nerve growth factor (Giannantoni et al. 2006b) and its receptors are involved in the pathophysiology of detrusor overactivity and bladder pain.

We believe that the necessary information has now been obtained for approval of BoNT treatment at least in patients with neurogenic detrusor overactivity. With regards to other applications, ongoing studies in well designed clinical trials will add a definite contribution to the preliminary results obtained in these pathologies.

Prof. Antonella Giannantoni, M.D., Ph.D.
Associate Professor of Urology
Department of Urology and Andrology
University of Perugia
Ospedale S. Maria della Misericordia
Perugia
Italy

11.8 Japan: Yukio Homma

Japan is now the most aged nation ever in the human history. Its urological relevance is increasing in both malignant and non-malignant urological diseases. Overactive bladder (OAB) is one of the typical non-malignant urological dysfunctions commonly diagnosed in the elderly. The national survey in 2002 indicated that 8.3 million Japanese suffer from OAB symptoms. Japanese people are opting for medical therapy for treatment of this condition; anticholinergics are the most common therapy for OAB. Secondary options such as electric and magnetic stimulation or bladder instillation are not popular. BoNT is expected as a novel option of significant efficacy for OAB refractory to conventional therapies.

The use of botulinum toxin is government-approved for torticollis but not for lower urinary tract dysfunction in Japan. Thus, we have experience with BoNT treatment only in investigational settings with a limited number of patients (Miyagawa et al. 2010). For neurogenic and non-neurogenic OAB, a dosage of 100–200 U of onabotulinumtoxinA is used. BoNT is injected at multiple submucosal or intra-detrusor sites of the bladder, sparing the trigone. Assessments include frequency-volume chart, uroflowmetry, residual urine measurement, and cytometry. Overactive Bladder Symptom Score (OABSS) (Homma et al. 2006), a sensitive score specific to OAB symptoms, is used for symptom assessment.

The efficacy we have observed thus far is promising with significant improvement in symptoms and urodynamic variables, confirming results from previous studies (Anger et al. 2010). While residual urine volume increased, urinary retention was rare. Another target of BoNT is interstitial cystitis and hypersensitive bladder syndrome (Homma et al. 2009). Our preliminary data suggests that injection of 100 U of onabotulinumtoxinA at the trigone relieves the pain and/or discomfort, which are characteristically associated with this condition. Interestingly the efficacy appears to be more pronounced for non-ulcer type interstitial cystitis and hypersensitive bladder syndrome. Injection into the sphincter muscle has also been attempted at few of our institutions.

Despite the rapid progress in urology, we have still many patients with intractable lower urinary tract dysfunction. BoNT injection has a high therapeutic potential for these conditions and we eagerly await the results of further clinical research. Basic research studies to elucidate the mechanisms of BoNT action or to develop an alternative to BoNT are also in progress. However, the regulation of pharmaceuticals is too strict for companies to do clinical trials and to apply for approval in Japan. Raising the research fund is the most crucial problem for Japanese investigators and patients, the potential beneficiary.

Professor Yukio Homma
Professor and Chairman
Department of Urology, Graduate School of Medicine
The University of Tokyo
Hongo 7-3-1, Bunkyoku
Tokyo, 113-8655
Japan

11.9   Korea: Kyu-Sung Lee

In Korea, botulinum toxin (BoNT) has been used since August 1995. BoNT is indicated for the treatment of strabismus and spasticity disorders. As for urology field, the use of BoNT is not approved for the lower urinary tract dysfunctions in Korea. However, we can use BoNT in investigational settings after the approval from institutional review boards and Korea Food and drug association. Currently BoNT are used for the treatment of lower urinary tract dysfunctions such as benign prostate hyperplasia (BPH), overactive bladder, interstitial cystitis, and chronic prostatitis/chronic pelvic pain syndrome refractory to conventional therapies in investigational settings.

In Korea, we have several articles for the use of BoNT. One study which was conducted in 2004, investigated the use of BoNT in detrusor external sphincter dyssynergia (Chung et al. 2005). A total of 100 units of onabotulinumtoxinA were injected at 4 sites, 3, 6, 9, and 12 o'clock relative to the external sphincter, under local anesthesia. At 1 month after the injection, the mean maximal flow rate was increased (from 8.4 to 12.2 ml/s) and mean residual urine was decreased (from 258 to 120 ml) compared to the baseline values. As a conclusion, transurethral BoNT injections were safe and effective for releasing or ameliorating a lower urinary tract obstruction due to detrusor sphincter dyssynergia. The study also reported that BoNT may be a safe and valuable therapeutic option in dyssynergic patients not desiring surgery or intermittent catheterization, and who are resistant to medications.

Another study evaluated the effect of BoNT for the treatment of BPH in 2004 (Park et al. 2006). Transperineal intraprostatic injection of onabotulinumtoxinA was carried out under transrectal ultrasonography. OnabotulinumtoxinA dissolved in 4–9 mL of saline was used from 100 to 300 U, according to prostate volume. Of 52 outpatients, 39 patients had subjective symptomatic relief at the 3 month follow-up. The storage symptoms were improved more than the voiding symptoms. Additionally, about 50% of the patients whose voiding symptom improved expressed improved erectile function. In summary, BoNT injection seems to be an alternative treatment for BPH.

Currently we are using BoNT as a new alternative option for lower urinary tract dysfunctions refractory to conventional therapies in investigational purpose. Many patients in Korea want minimal invasive treatment. And polypharmacy is common and bother some to the patients. Many patients of old age take 3–5 class of medication for the control of chronic disease and want to reduce the number of drug. Despite potential urologic applications of BoNT, more studies including economic outcome are necessary for the approval of BoNT in Korea.

Kyu-Sung Lee, M.D., Ph.D.
Professor
Department of Urology, Samsung Medical Center
Sungkyunkwan University School of Medicine
General Director, Division of Clinical Trial Training, Clinical Trial Center
Samsung Medical Center
Korea

11.10 The Netherlands: John Heesakkers

Two types of botulinum toxin A are available in the Netherlands: onabotulinumtoxinA (Botox, Allergan, Inc., Irvine, CA) and abobotulinumtoxinA (Dysport; Ipsen Ltd., Berkshire, UK). The first Dutch urological applications were explored in 2001 and published about in 2003 during the annual spring meeting of the Dutch Urological Association by Balk and associates. The indication was urodynamically proven idiopathic detrusor overactivity. The product used was abobotulinumtoxinA and the injections were given under general anesthesia at 25 places with 20 U of abobotulinumtoxinA injected at each site. The population consisted of 15 patients that were followed-up for a mean of 136 (range 47–430) days. The mean cystometric capacity went up from 228 to 433 ml. Daily voiding frequency was reduced from 14 to 9 episodes per day. Three patients (20%) had a residual urine volume of greater than 100 ml and had to begin intermittent self catheterization. Delaere and associates subsequently reported a lower risk of retention of less than 10%.

Initially, intradetrusor injections were given under general or regional anesthesia, but soon it appeared that it was feasible to do the procedure under local anesthesia.

We presented at the International Continence Society in 2009 our study on improved pain scores with BoNT with 10 injections under local anesthesia.

Nowadays BoNT in the Netherlands is widely used in many urological clinics as well as university clinics. The most frequent indication is idiopathic or neurogenic overactive bladder or detrusor overactivity. There is some experience with bladder pain syndrome and radiation cystitis but data is scarce.

The cost of the injected material is categorized in the "expensive drugs" class. This implies that 75% of every used vial, that has to be covered by the hospital budget, is reimbursed by the national health system. In 2011 there still is no proper reimbursement policy for the complete treatment including hospital and doctor's fee. In the Netherlands patients do not pay partially or completely for whatever medical treatment so no possibilities exist to correct for the above mentioned inconvenience. The treatment of detrusor overactivity or overactive bladder with botulinum toxin is not yet registered in the Netherlands yet. However, since the treatment of overactive bladder and detrusor overactivity with BoNT injections is mentioned as a proven treatment in many international guidelines, it is not very difficult to offer BoNT injections to patients without a lot of administrative paperwork.

Professor John Heesakkers
Department of Urology
Radboud University Nijmegen MC
The Netherlands

11.11 Portugal: Francisco Cruz

In Portugal, botulinum toxin application into the lower urinary tract started in the beginning of this century, soon after the first reports on the topic. Like in other countries, BoNT was initially used as a treatment for urinary incontinence caused by neurogenic detrusor overactivity refractory to standard management. Being at that time an off-label treatment, its application was dependent upon a specific authorization of the ethics committee of each institution.

The simplicity of BoNT application, the total dose of onabotulinumtoxinA, 200–300 U or abobotulinumtoxinA, 500–750 U being divided by 30 injections of 1 ml each in the detrusor wall turned this treatment extremely attractive for the treatment of neurogenic detrusor overactivity not adequately managed by antimuscarinics. The efficacy of the treatment can also be attested by the reduced number of bladder augmentations being performed nowadays in neurogenic detrusor overactivity patients. No severe adverse events associated with the treatment were reported in this country.

Since 2005 urinary incontinence caused by idiopathic detrusor overactivity refractory to antimuscarinic drugs also became an indication for BoNT injections. As in neurogenic detrusor overactivity cases, an authorization from ethics committee is necessary. Fewer centers are using this treatment when compared with neurogenic detrusor overactivity management. Nevertheless our personal experience with onabotulinumtoxinA, 100 U injected in 30 sites of the bladder wall is very satisfactory, the treatment being highly effective for controlling urinary incontinence while causing a low rate of urinary retention.

Our center is presently investigating BoNT in two other lower urinary tract conditions, BPH, and bladder pain syndrome/interstitial cystitis. A low number of cases, refractory to standard treatment have been treated. For the first indication onabotulinumtoxinA 100 U are injected in each transitional zone of the prostate. For pain syndrome/interstitial cystitis, onabotulinumtoxinA 100 U injections are restricted to the trigonal area of the bladder to maximize nociceptive fiber intoxication and to minimize the risk of voiding dysfunction.

Professor Francisco Cruz
Professor and Chairman of Urology
Hospital de São João and Faculty of Medicine of Porto
Porto
Portugal

11.12 Singapore: Michael Wong

The application of BoNT in Urology has seen a steady rise in the last 5 years in Singapore. To date, its main usage has been to manage refractory idiopathic overactive bladder, neurogenic bladder hyperactivity in spinal injury patients and bladder-neck dyssynergia.

One of the interesting aspects of Singapore healthcare is that for the most part long-term paraplegic patients with bladder issues are managed in one hospital (Tan Tock Seng Hospital) which has specialized and dedicated neurological services. This arrangement limits urological experience of management in this particular group of patients to a few in-house urologists (Tow et al. 2007) who started using BoNT in 2004. This trend will continue to move forward. At the same time, two other academic urological centers initiated BoNT trials (Lim and Quek 2008; Lie et al. 2010) in 2004 and this was the catalyst for its subsequent increased usage. BoNT usage in the private sector only started at Mount Elizabeth Hospital in 2007 but has seen limited growth to date.

In my opinion, the usage of BoNT to treat benign prostatic hyperplasia will be limited due to a particular strength of the Singapore urology residency program where one would be expected to complete nearly 100 bipolar transurethral prostatectomies by the end of one's residency. This will result in a limited enthusiasm for other minimally invasive options like BoNT injectable and even laser prostatectomy option. On the other hand, the growth of BoNT in both bladder and bladder neck pathology will be expected to increase in the coming years.

Dr. Michael Y.C. Wong
President of Singapore Urology Association
Medical Director of Singapore Urology and Fertility Centre at Mount Elizabeth
Mount Elizabeth Medical Centre #10-09
Singapore 228510

11.13 Taiwan: Alex T.L. Lin

The concept of using botulinum toxin (BoNT) to treat functional disorders of the lower urinary tract was first introduced into Taiwan by Dr. Chancellor in 2001. He gave a talk in the annual meeting of Taiwan Urological Association held in Kaohsiung, a southern city where Dr. Chancellor stayed during his childhood. His revolutionary concept much impressed Taiwanese urologists. Only Professor HC Kuo in Hualien was brave enough to carry out clinical trials and demonstrated the effectiveness of the BoNT on many difficult cases with voiding dysfunction. Dr. Yao-Chi Chuang in Kaohsiung also confirmed the efficacy of BoNT by multiple clinical and laboratory research studies. Their achievements were well known quickly throughout the island via public media.

People in Taiwan possess an adventurous character and quite comfortably accept new things. Many patients went to their urologists requesting BoNT treatment even though it's a toxin. The needs from the patients prompted the Taiwanese Continence Society to deliver educational courses to local urologists. For international communication, in 2006 the Taiwan Continence Society organized an international symposium in Taipei and a workshop in the Annual Meeting of International Continence Society in Christchurch. Now BoNT injection is a regular treatment option for voiding dysfunction in the majority of medical centers in Taiwan. BoNT is not yet approved for the use in the lower urinary tract in Taiwan. According to the law, patients have to be informed that BoNT usage in the lower urinary tract is off-label and this consent has to be documented in the medical record. The National Health Insurance, which enrolls 98% of the Taiwanese population, does not cover the cost and patients have to pay. But many patients are still willing to pay for the treatment.

Accumulating observations from clinical experiences and bench studies from Taiwan and other parts of the world have confirmed the safety and efficacy of BoNT injection in treating voiding dysfunction. Although BoNT is not good enough for all types of voiding dysfunction, it does provide effective rescue for some patients who have no option. I fully believe that with time and through more clinical and lab research, using BoNT and other neurotoxins will evolve to be one of standard treatments for voiding dysfunction in all parts of the world.

Alex T.L. Lin, M.D., Ph.D.
President, Taiwanese Continence Society, 2000–2006.
Professor and Chief
Department of Urology
Taipei Veterans General Hospital
National Yang Ming University
Taipei
Taiwan

11.14 United Kingdom: Arun Sahai and Prokar Dasgupta

Botulinum toxin treatment has revolutionised the treatment of refractory overactive bladder. The United Kingdom has contributed significantly to the published literature in advancing this treatment to where it is today. Initial use in the UK was with Professor Dasgupta and Professor Fowler at the National Hospital for Neurology and Neurosurgery. There the "Dasgupta technique" for administration as an outpatient procedure under local anaesthetic was developed and is the favoured method employed by the majority of clinicians. The first randomised controlled trial in the use of botulinum toxin in idiopathic detrusor overactivity was conducted at Guy's Hospital, London demonstrating improved symptoms, urodynamics, and quality of life for these patients.

Apostolos Apostlidis, working at Queen Square, was interested in the toxins' mechanism of action in the bladder and demonstrated its effectiveness in down regulating human afferent receptors implicated in detrusor overactivity. He also put forward a complex hypothesis as to its combined mechanism of action working on both motor and sensory components to the bladder. Repeated injections of botulinum toxin have also been reported as safe and effective in treating neurogenic and idiopathic detrusor overactivity for up to 9 years.

In the UK patients are treated on either a named patient basis or in clinical trials. Some of the largest contributors to the Phase II and III international trials of the toxin were from the UK. We have also reported on its cost-effectiveness and it is now recognised in the National Institute of Clinical Excellence (NICE, 2006) guidelines for urinary incontinence as a second line treatment for those who have failed conservative treatment and medical therapy. However as the product is unlicensed, hospital trusts are sometimes unwilling to fund its use.

Drs Chancellor and Smith are to be congratulated for writing this book. Both are experts in the field and have contributed significantly to bringing this treatment into mainstream clinical practice and to understanding its complex mechanism of action.

Arun Sahai, F.R.C.S. (Urol), Ph.D., B.Sc. (Hons.)
Specialist Trainee and NIHR Academic Clinical Lecturer in Urology
Prokar Dasgupta, M.Sc. (Urol), M.D., D.L.S., F.R.C.S. (Urol), F.E.B.U.
Professor of Urological Innovation and Hon. Consultant Urological Surgeon
Urology Department
MRC Centre for Transplantation
Guy's Hospital, King's College London
London
UK

11.15 United Kingdom Urogynaecology: Anga S. Arunkalaivanan

Botulinum toxin type A is the most studied of the serotypes available and it is this serotype that has found therapeutic use. The minimal invasiveness of this toxin injection in the bladder makes it attractive in the treatment of refractory detrusor overactivity. It is usually performed using a rigid cystoscope in a day-case or inpatient setting and a flexible cystoscope in an outpatient setting. However, flexible cystoscopic injection of botulinum toxin done under local anesthetic has the added advantages of good tolerability and cost effectiveness. Botulinum toxin type A received National Institute of Clinical Excellence (NICE, UK) approval for the treatment of intractable detrusor overactivity in 2006 although it is still not licensed.

Initially there have been concerns about the safety, long term efficacy, etc. However, a European consensus report has given a grade A recommendation for the use of botulinum toxin-A in the treatment of overactive bladder syndrome and idiopathic detrusor overactivity (Apostolidis et al. 2009). Sahai and colleagues (2007) report that repeated injections with BoNT in patients with IDO are safe.

The uses of botulinum toxin in urogynaecology have expanded to include detrusor sphincter dyssynergia and interstitial cystitis. Nevertheless, the evidence from the studies thus far suggests a trend towards short-term benefit with intravesical BoNT injections in refractory interstitial cystitis, but further robust evidence is required.

Recently, there have been a number of potential applications in gynecology which include vaginismus, vestibulodynia, and chronic pelvic pain. Botulinum toxin was first described for the treatment of vaginismus in a case report published in The Lancet in 1997. Since then, a few more studies confirmed its use in this patient population. This appears to be the most promising of the alternative gynecological uses of botulinum toxin.

For vestibulodynia, there are limited data, in the form of case reports and small series, to indicate that BoNT injections may provide short-term (3–6 months) benefit (Abbott et al. 2006). Retreatment is reported to be successful and side effects are few. Class-I studies are essential to adequately assess this form of treatment.

Although the use of BoNT in idiopathic and neurogenic detrusor overactivity is now well proven and widely accepted, its use in other potential gynaecological conditions is in its infancy. In these conditions, further research and clinical trials are required before BoNT can be recommended in routine clinical practice.

Anga S. Arunkalaivanan, M.D., F.R.C.O.G.
Honorary Senior Lecturer (University of Birmingham)
Consultant Urogynaecologist and Obstetrician
City Hospital
Dudley Road
Birmingham B18 7QH
UK

References

Canada: Sender Herschorn

Canadian Institute for Health Information (2010) National Health Expenditure Trends, 1975 to 2010. CIHI, Ottawa, ON

Corcos J, Schick E (2004) Prevalence of overactive bladder and incontinence in Canada. Can J Urol 11:2278–2284

Herschorn S, Gajewski J, Schulz J, Corcos J (2008) A population-based study of urinary symptoms and incontinence: the Canadian urinary bladder survey. BJU Int 101:52–58

Milsom I, Irwin DE (2007) A cross-sectional, population-based multinational study of the prevalence of overactive badder and lower urinary tract symptoms: results from the EPIC study. Eur Urol Suppl 6:4–9

Italy: Antonella Giannantoni

Giannantoni A, Costantini E, Di Stasi SM, Tascini MC, Bini V, Porena M (2006a) Botulinum A toxin intravesical injections in the treatment of painful bladder syndrome: a pilot study. Eur Urol 49:704–709

Giannantoni A, Di Stasi SM, Nardicchi V, Zucchi A, Macchioni L, Bini V, Goracci G, Porena M (2006b) Botulinum-A toxin injections into the detrusor muscle decrease nerve growth factor bladder tissue levels in patients with neurogenic detrusor overactivity. J Urol 175:2341–2344

Maria G, Brisinda G, Civello IM, Bentivoglio AR, Sganga G, Albanese A (2003) Relief by botulinum toxin of voiding dysfunction due to benign prostatic hyperplasia: results of a randomized, placebo-controlled study. Urology 62:259–264

Schurch B, Stohrer M, Kramer G, Schmid DM, Gaul G, Hauri D (2000) Botulinum-A toxin for treating detrusor hyperreflexia in spinal cord injured patients: a new alternative to anticholinergic drugs? Preliminary results. J Urol 164:692–697

Japan: Yukio Homma

Anger JT, Weinberg A, Suttorp MJ et al (2010) Outcomes of intravesical botulinum toxin for idiopathic overactive bladder symptoms: a systematic review of the literature. J Urol 183:2258–2264

Homma Y, Yoshida M, Seki N et al (2006) Symptom assessment tool for overactive bladder syndrome – overactive bladder symptom score. Urology 68:318–323

Homma Y, Ueda T, Tomoe H et al (2009) Clinical guidelines for interstitial cystitis and hypersensitive bladder syndrome. Int J Urol 16:597–615

Miyagawa I, Watanabe T, Isoyama T, Honda M et al (2010) Experience with injections of botulinum toxin type A into the detrusor muscle. Aktuelle Urol 41:S24–S26

Korea: Kyu-Sung Lee

Chung KJ et al (2005) The efficacy of botulinum toxin injection to the external urethral sphincter for detrusor external sphincter dyssynergia Korean. J Urol 46:604–609

Park DS et al (2006) Evaluation of short term clinical effects and presumptive mechanism of botulinum toxin type A as a treatment modality of benign prostatic hyperplasia. Yonsei Med J 47:706–714

Singapore: Michael Wong

Lie KY, Wong MY, Ng LG (2010) Botulinum toxin A for idiopathic detrusor overactivity. Ann Acad Med Singapore 39:714–715

Lim SK, Quek PL (2008) Intraprostatic and bladder-neck injection of Botulinum A toxin in treatment of males with bladder-neck dyssynergia: a pilot study. Eur Urol 53:620–625

Tow AM, Toh KL, Pang SP, Consigliere D (2007) Botulinum toxin type A for refractory detrusor overactivity in spinal cord injured patients in Singapore. Ann Acad Med Singapore 36:11–17

United Kingdom Urogynaecology: Anga S. Arunkalaivanan

Abbott JA, Jarvis SK, Lyons SD, Thomson A, Vancaille TG (2006) Botulinum toxin type A for chronic pain and pelvic floor spasm in women: a randomized controlled trial. Obstet Gynecol 108:915–923

Apostolidis A, Dasgupta P, Denys P et al (2009) Recommendations on the use of botulinum toxin in the treatment of lower urinary tract disorders and pelvic floor dysfunctions: a European consensus report. Eur Urol 55:100–119

National Institute of Clinical Excellence (2006). http://www.nice.org.uk/

Sahai A, Dowson C, Khan MS, Dasguta P, GKTBS Group (2007) Repeated injections of botulinum toxin-A for idiopathic detrusor overactivity. Urology 75:552–558

Appendix 1

Patient Instruction for Botulinum Toxin Bladder Injection

NOTE: If you usually take oral antibiotics prior to dental appointments, we would like you to do the same before the bladder injection treatment session. If you have any questions please check with your cardiologist.

NOTE: Please remember that you may need to limit taking medications that affect bleeding prior to treatment. This includes aspirin, warfarin and ibuprofen products. Please speak to us directly before procedure about this. If you have taken such medicine please inform the nurse as soon as possible.

- As this is an office procedure performed solely with local anesthesia, it is not necessary for you to have someone drive you home. If your procedure is being done in the operating room as other procedures are also necessary, please note you will receive some sedation prior to examination and treatment and will require someone to drive you home per hospital protocols.
- You are allowed to eat and drink the morning of your treatment.

The Day of Treatment Session

NOTE: Please update your doctor about any new medications or other therapies. We would like to know about prescription medicines, over the counter medications, as well as any herbal/alternative remedies. Please bring a list of all your known medication allergies.

- The day of your treatment, you will be asked to take a single dose of oral antibiotic to prevent a urine infection. Please take the prescribed antibiotic 1 h before your scheduled treatment.
- Once you have been comfortably positioned on the procedure bed, the genital area will be washed and draped.
- A soft rubber catheter will be lubricated and inserted to drain the bladder empty of urine. Then, before removing the same catheter, numbing liquid [1% lidocaine] will be pushed through the catheter into the bladder. No needles are used for this process to numb your bladder.
- After the numbing solution sits for 15 min, it will be drained and your doctor will proceed with the treatment.

Fig. 1 Dr. Chancellor with flexible cystoscope

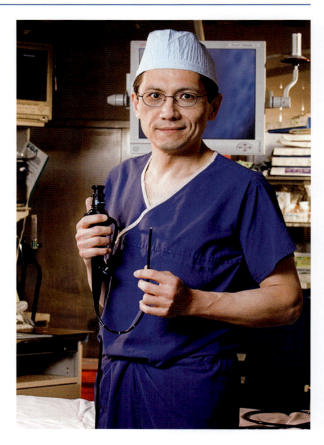

The cystoscope [camera type device] is guided into the bladder, allowing your doctor to inject the botulinum toxin medicine into the bladder wall. Fig. 1 this injection process will take approximately 15 min to complete.

After the treatment is finished, you will be asked to remain in the clinic for at least 30 min for observation. Also, we will ask that you urinate before leaving the office.

If you are unable to urinate to empty your bladder [urinary retention], your doctor may want you to use a temporary catheter to drain the bladder.

What to Expect After Treatment

- You may notice some pain in your pelvic and/or bladder area; some blood-tinged urine, as well as possible difficulty urinating. These symptoms should resolve within 24 h. Otherwise, please inform your doctor's office if you note: Fever > 101°F

Inability to urinate
Blood without urine
- The botulinum toxin medication will not work instantly. It may take several days or weeks to notice a gradual improvement in overactive bladder symptoms.
- Please continue all overactive bladder medications for at least 2 weeks.

Risks of Treatment

Potential risks include bleeding, infection and urinary retention. If urinary retention occurs, meaning you cannot empty your bladder, you may need to begin self-catheterization. This requires that you would place a tiny soft tube into your bladder several times per day to empty your bladder as it has become too relaxed to empty on its own.

In addition, all botulinum toxin formulations must contain a Black Box Warning mandated by the FDA. Here is the Black Box Warning for onabotulinumtoxinA (Botox®, Allergan, Inc., Irvine, CA):

BOTOX® and BOTOX® Cosmetic may cause serious side effects that can be life threatening. Call your doctor or get medical help right away if you have any of these problems after treatment with BOTOX® or BOTOX® Cosmetic:
- Problems swallowing, speaking, or breathing. These problems can happen hours to weeks after an injection of BOTOX® or BOTOX® Cosmetic usually because the muscles that you use to breathe and swallow can become weak after the injection. Death can happen as a complication if you have severe problems with swallowing or breathing after treatment with BOTOX® or BOTOX® Cosmetic.
- Swallowing problems may last for several months. People who already have swallowing or breathing problems before receiving BOTOX® or BOTOX® Cosmetic have the highest risk of getting these problems.
- Spread of toxin effects. In some cases, the effect of botulinum toxin may affect areas of the body away from the injection site and cause symptoms of a serious condition called botulism. The symptoms of botulism include: loss of strength and muscle weakness all over the body, double vision, blurred vision and drooping eyelids, hoarseness or change or loss of voice (dysphonia), trouble saying words clearly (dysarthria), loss of bladder control, trouble breathing, trouble swallowing.

Appendix 2

Patient Instruction for Botulinum Toxin Prostate Injection

If you usually take oral antibiotics prior to dental appointments we would ask you to do the same before this procedure. If you have any questions please check with your cardiologist.

If you are taking medications that affect bleeding prior to treatment, including aspirin, warfare in or ibuprofen products, please be off the medication for at least 5 days before the procedure. If you cannot be off the medications for that long please speak to us and your medical doctor as to alternative treatments. If you have accidentally taken such medicine immediately prior to procedure, please inform a staff member as soon as possible.

This injection is done in our office using an anesthetic and general takes less than 30 min to complete. The procedure consists of using a needle to inject botulinum toxin into the prostate. You are allowed to eat and drink the morning or afternoon of your treatment. You will be able to drive yourself after the procedure.

The Day of Treatment Session

Please update your doctor about any new medications or other therapies. We would like to know about prescription medicines, over the counter medications, as well as any herbal/nutraceutical remedies.

- The morning of the procedure please use an enema to cleanse the bowel.
- The day of your treatment, you will be asked to take a single dose of oral antibiotic to prevent infection. Please take the prescribed medication at least 1 h prior to your appointment.
- During the procedure you will be positioned on your left side with your legs curled toward your abdomen.
- The ultrasound probe is placed into the rectum and the prostate is viewed.
- The injection needle is placed through the probe and the botulinum is injected into each side of the prostate.
- After the treatment is finished, you will be asked to remain in the clinic for at least 30 min for observation. We will ask that you urinate before leaving the office.

What to Expect After Treatment

- You may notice some pain in your prostate or bladder area; some blood-tinged urine or semen for several days. You should not have difficulty urinating.
- The botulinum toxin medication will not work instantly. It may take several days or weeks to notice changes in your urination patterns. Please continue the use of all medications for at least 2 weeks.

Appendix 3

Nursing Care of the Patient Receiving Botulinum Toxin

Nurses play an important role in the direct care experience in patients considering botulinum toxin treatment of the urinary tract. The nurse is ideally placed to provide education regarding the specific treatment, the procedure, expected outcomes, potential side effects, and assessment of effectiveness.

Pre-procedure

The nurse should assist in the screening of appropriate patients for this treatment and may be the main provider of pre- and postoperative teaching and follow-up. Initially, the dose based on intended outcomes must be determined for each patient by the physician. Patients must also be assessed prior to the procedure for their willingness to perform intermittent catheterization as there is a risk of urinary retention. Patients who may be unwilling or physically unable to perform catheterizations may not be suitable candidates.

Prior authorization should take place before any surgical arrangements are made as decisions may take several days to weeks. It is important to not place undo financial hardship on a patient who may not be able to afford part or all of the procedure and/or medication cost. Facilities may need to purchase and bill the medication, or have the patient be responsible for purchasing the BoNT, if the treatment will not be reimbursed.

Prior to the procedure, providers may choose to order a urinalysis, urine culture, and sensitivity testing so that any underlying medical problems are identified. Depending upon the patient and symptoms, antibiotics may be ordered to treat an infection. Gentamycin is not recommended as a form of treatment for infection or prophylaxis due to the potential risk of neuromuscular blockade.

Extra care should be taken in patients on anticoagulant therapies. Aspirin may need to be discontinued 7–10 days prior to the procedure. Patients who are on oral warfarin should stop the medication 5 days prior to procedure. If they are unable to temporarily discontinue the medication, one may need to be switched to a subcutaneously administered anticoagulant for several days prior to the procedure. Warfarin can typically be resumed the evening after the injections.

To minimize the potential risk of pain in an office setting when no general anesthesia or intravenous sedation is used, it is suggested that lidocaine (1% or 2%, 20–40 mL) be placed into the bladder 15–20 min prior to the procedure. Prior to the injections, the lidocaine is drained from the bladder. Care should be taken to place patients in a comfortable position, especially patients who complain of muscle spasticity, so that pain in the extremities and back can be avoided.

Preparing Botulinum Toxin

Onabotulinumtoxin A will be used as an example due to our vast experience with this product. Prior to injection, vacuum-dried onabotulinumtoxinA (Allergan, Inc., Irvine, CA), which appears as a very small amount of opaque, dried particulate within the small clear bottle, must be reconstituted with sterile, preservative-free normal saline according to the prescribing information. The diluent should be drawn up in the appropriate size syringe and slowly injected into the onabotulinumtoxinA vial. The contents should then be gently mixed by rotating the vial. Do not shake the vial. Reconstituted onabotulinumtoxinA should be clear, colorless, and free of particulate matter.

The date and time of reconstitution should be recorded on the label in the space provided. OnabotulinumtoxinA should be administered within 24 h after reconstitution. Once reconstituted, onabotulinumtoxinA should be stored in a refrigerator at 2–8°C (36–46°F).

As with all injectable products, reconstituted onabotulinumtoxinA should be inspected visually for particulate matter and discoloration prior to administration. An injection of onabotulinumtoxinA is prepared by drawing slightly more than the intended dose of the properly reconstituted toxin into an appropriate size sterile syringe. A new, sterile needle and syringe should be used each time onabotulinumtoxinA is drawn from the vial. If not all of the medication is used the amount discarded must be recorded in the patient record.

Medication Information on OnabotulinumtoxinA

Contraindications: OnabotulinumtoxinA is contraindicated in the presence of infection at the proposed injection site(s) and in individuals with known hypersensitivity to any botulinum toxin preparation or to any of the components in the formulation.

Drug interactions: Co-administration of onabotulinumtoxinA and aminoglycosides (gentamycin) or other agents interfering with neuromuscular transmission (such as curare compounds) should only be performed with caution because the effect of the toxin might be potentiated.

Adverse reactions: Allergan (2009) has added a black box warning to their label and per Federal Drug Administration (FDA) requirements patients must be given a medication guide each time onabotulinumtoxinA is administered. Adverse reactions are related to the location of the injection and are rare with urological procedures. The main concerns with urinary tract injection are infection and urinary retention.

Dosage: The dosage will be determined by the physician based on each patient but is usually 100–300 U onabotulinumtoxinA. We typically use 100 U onabotulinumtoxinA for idiopathic and 200 U onabotulinumtoxinA for neurogenic overactive bladder.

Injection Procedures

Ten milliliter of preservative-free saline is typically used to dilute every 100 U onabotulinumtoxinA vial, and the injection volume is typically 0.5–1.0 mL at each injection site. Injection needles used in urology are typically 22–27 gauge and 4–8mm long.

Botulinum toxin can be injected using a rigid or flexible scope, depending on patient or surgeon preference. Rigid systems allow for quicker, more controllable injections, whereas flexible scopes are generally more comfortable for patients, especially men. Patients with a spinal cord injury may experience discomfort during the procedure, depending upon injury level and severity of muscle spasticity.

Post-procedure

Pain is a rare but potential symptom that may occur as a result of the injection process, lasting minutes to several hours after the procedure. This usually occurs only in patients with a history of a bladder pain syndrome or patients who admit to neuropathic pain. Patients may be directed to use over the counter products such as acetaminophen for pain.

Hematuria may occur during the procedure but should be minimal upon completion of the procedure. Patients need to be instructed that if any clotting occurs after the procedure, the physician should be notified immediately. These complications are rare, but can occur and should be discussed with the patient or caregiver prior to treatment.

Rates of retention and subsequent need for intermittent catheterization vary considerably between studies depending on the dosage and medical issues of the patient. Retention may be intended based on the underlying condition. For example, complete continence with retention is a highly positive outcome in a spinal cord injured patient already performing self-catheterization. In contrast, retention would be a negative outcome in an ambulatory woman with idiopathic overactive bladder and rare urgency incontinence. Prior to the procedure, all patients must be informed and trained in self-catheterization.

All patients, but especially those with a history of infections, should be instructed to watch for any signs and symptoms of infection, including fever, chills, cloudy urine, blood in the urine, painful urination, and new or increasing incontinence symptoms.

The onset of effectiveness of BoNT can vary from a noticeable change within several days to a more slow insidious effect over 4–6 week. Patients should be instructed to monitor urinary frequency and urine flow as well as abdominal girth. Patients with neurogenic urinary dysfunction who pre-procedure does not perform intermittent catheterization and is receiving a higher dose of onabotulinumtoxinA (i.e., 200 U) should be provided with equipment and a system to monitor their voiding schedules.

Repeated Injections

Patients should initially return to the office within 2–4 weeks of treatment so that efficacy can be determined, retention assessed, and catheterization schedules reviewed in those who perform intermittent catheterization.

Repeat injections of BoNT can be used to provide ongoing efficacy, but re-injection of BoNT should not be performed sooner than every 3 months due to the potential risk of developing neutralizing antibodies and subsequent treatment resistance. If a patient has received BoNT to another area of the body (e.g., for lower limb spasticity or cosmetic purposes), it may be prudent to combine both injections within a 24 h window or, alternatively, to space all injections at least 3 months apart. Risk factors for antibody formation include short intervals between injections, booster injections when optimal efficacy is not initially achieved, increasing doses at each injection, and a high cumulative dose. The development of antibodies against BoNT, according to recent evidence, appears to be less that 1.0% in licensed indications.

Impact on Quality of Life

Symptom scales and diaries are useful for evaluating the effectiveness of BoNT treatments. Using these tools, patients can easily provide an overall evaluation of symptom response using a measurement tool such as a visual analog scale. Symptoms such as frequency, incontinence, and nocturia should specifically be evaluated before and 6–8 weeks after treatments, and then as needed in order to capture important clinical data which may be required for future treatments and reimbursement.

As bladder symptoms improve with treatment, especially if symptoms improve gradually over weeks or months, patients may forget previous voiding patterns such as frequency and nocturia. Prior evaluations and diaries can help to demonstrate improvement to patients as well as to motivate them to continue with effective therapies. This may be important information to provide to insurance companies to support the need for either initial or repeated injections.

Index

A
Acetylcholine, 14, 20, 62, 92
Achalasia, 159, 160
Adverse reactions, 202
Afferents, 22
Alpha antagonists, 72, 112, 115, 123, 132
5-Alpha reductase inhibitors, 112, 115, 123
Aminoglycosides, 118, 202
Anal fissure, 159, 161, 162
Antibiotics, 117, 195, 199, 201
Antibody, 23, 43, 204
Anticholinergic, 68
Anticoagulant therapies, 201
Antitoxin, 5
ATP, 92
Augmentation, 38, 76, 102, 169, 170, 172, 173, 182
Australia, 177
Autonomic dysreflexia, 33, 142
Autonomic hyperfunction, 164
Axonal sprouting, 22

B
BCG cystitis, 90
Belgium, 178
Biofeedback, 146
Biological activity, 38
Black box warning, 196
Bladder
  base, 39
  dome, 39
  fibrosis, 48
  inflammation, 20
Bladder neck dyssynergia, 147
Blepharospasm, 14
Botox, 8
Botulism, 5, 36, 197
BPH, 111, 164, 182, 186

C
Canada, 179
Capsaicin, 61
Cerebral palsy, 32, 96, 166
Cervical cancer, 146
Cervical dystonia, 5, 14, 83
CGRP, 21, 62, 92
Clostridium botulinum, 5
Compliance, 95, 106
Conservative therapy, 106
Contraindications, 202
Cost-effectiveness ratio, 173
CP/CPPS, 90
Cumulative cost, 171
Cystoscope, 36, 37, 62, 63

D
Depth of injection, 100
Detrusor pressure, 44, 104
Detrusor-sphincter dyssynergia (DSD), 29, 105, 131
Diluent, 202
Disulfide bond, 15
Drooling, 165, 166
Drug interactions, 202
Duration of effect, 47
Dysarthria, 3
Dysfunctional voider, 135
Dysmenorrhea, 148
Dyspareunia, 148
Dysphonia, 3
Dysport, 9

E
Electromyography (EMG), 7, 34, 138, 142
Enterocystoplasty, 177
Epididymitis, 127, 128
Esophagus, 160

European panel of experts, 71
Evidence based, 144

F
Flow rate, 124
Formulation, 23
France, 180

G
Gabapentin, 126
Gastroparesis, 159
Generic equivalents, 8
Gentamycin, 202
Germany, 181
Glabellar lines, 83
Glutamate, 62, 158, 159

H
Headache, 158
Health economics, 169–174
Hematuria, 127, 204
Hydronephrosis, 98, 105
Hyperalgesia, 24
Hyperhidrosis, 14, 156, 163
    axillary, 164, 165
    palmar, 163, 165
Hypertonic pelvic floor, 148

I
Idiopathic overactive bladder,
    20, 22, 39, 63, 64, 72,
    73, 100, 179, 181, 203
Immunogenicity, 11
India, 181
Infection, 128, 203
Inflammatory cystitis, 90
Intermittent catheterization, 201, 204
Internalization of toxin, 15
Internal sphincter dyssynergia, 143, 147
Interstitial cystitis/painful bladder syndrome
    (IC/PBS), 80, 84, 182, 188
Intramuscular, 64
Italy, 183

J
Japan, 184

K
Korea, 185

L
Lethal dose, 9
Levator ani, 148, 149
Lidocaine, 62, 82, 144, 195
Local anesthesia, 72

M
Markov decision analysis, 172
Mast cell, 92
Meta-analysis, 69
Migraine, 158
Modified injection technique, 63
MRI, 39, 40, 64
Multiple sclerosis, 30
Multi-specialty interactions, 10
Muscarinic receptors, 20
Myelodysplasia, 32, 95, 99
Myelomeningocele, 96, 101
Myobloc, 10

N
National Institute of Health and Clinical
    Excellence (NICE), 174, 191
Netherlands, 186
Neurobloc, 10
Neurogenic detrusor overactivity, 29
Neuromodulation, 76, 150
Neuropeptides, 20
Neutralizing antibodies, 23
NGF, 22
Nitroglycerin, 162
Nocturnal enuresis, 147
Non-neurogenic, 138, 145
Norepinephrine, 92
Nursing care, 201

O
Off-label, 66
Overactive bladder, 24
Overactive bladder symptom score
    (OABSS), 184

P
Pain, 155
    back pain, 156
    genital pain, 148
    headache, 158
    male chronic pelvic pain syndrome, 79, 90
    myofascial pain syndromes, 156, 157
    painful levator syndrome, 134
    pelvic pain, 79, 134, 149

Paralysis, 39, 41
Parkinson's disease, 32
Pediatric, 38, 95, 105
Pelvic floor disorders 134
Pelvic prolapse, 81
Percutaneous tibial nerve stimulation, 174
Periurethral, 137, 141
Pooled analysis, 70
Portugal, 187
Potency, 5, 8
Prostate, 113, 164
  atrophy, 113
  apoptosis, 114
  biopsy, 116, 118, 122, 123
  cancer, 116
  median lobe enlargement, 116
Prostatitis, 79, 112, 116, 121, 126, 127, 149
PSA, 112, 116, 124
Ptosis, 4
Pubococcygeus muscles, 90, 140, 148
Puborectalis muscles, 90, 147
Pubovaginal sling, 147
Pudendal nerve block, 82, 86, 139, 149
Pyloric sphincter 162

Q
Quality of life, 69

R
Radiation cystitis, 90
Reconstitution, 37, 117, 137, 202
Rehabilitation, 7
Repeat injection, 47, 106
Residual urine, 69, 72, 124
Resiniferatoxin, 56, 61
Retrograde ejaculation, 128, 146
Risk-benefit ratio, 73, 76

S
Sacral neuromodulation, 57, 76, 169, 170
Salivary glands, 164
Sausage poison, 13
Self-catheterization, 72, 85, 141, 196
Senory neurons, 79
Shy-bladder syndrome, 133, 135
Simultaneous bladder and sphincter injection, 41, 55, 145
Singapore, 188
Smooth muscle, 161
SNAP–25, 17
SNARE, 16, 17, 24
Spasticity, 3

Sphincter, 106, 131, 137
  endoluminal stent, 133
  sphincterotomy, 133
  sphincter spasm, 161
Spina bifida, 96
Spinal cord injury, 30
Spinal needle, 43
Storage, 117
Strabismus, 14
Stress urinary incontinence, 90, 144
Submucosa, 64, 101
Substance P, 21, 62, 92
Suburothelium, 39, 40, 84, 100
Sweat glands, 164, 165
Synaptic vesicle protein (SV2), 17
Synaptobrevin, 17
Syntaxin, 17

T
Taiwan, 189
Tethered cord, 96
Trabeculation, 99
Transient receptor potential channel vanilloid family member 1 (TRPV1), 21
Translocation, 15
Transrectal ultrasound, 137
Treatment cost, 171
Trigone, 39, 41, 62, 63, 66, 71, 76, 84, 88, 101
Trigone-sparing, 62

U
Ultrasound, 118, 123, 128, 199
United Kingdom, 190
Urinary retention, 35, 39, 111, 196
Urinary tract infection, 111
Urodynamic, 33, 44, 47, 71

V
Vaccine, 6
Vaginismus, 134
Vesicoureteral reflux, 31, 40, 62, 84, 98, 101, 104
Voiding dysfunction, 105
Vulva, 85
Vulvodynia, 6, 141, 149

W
Warfarin, 195, 201

X
Xeomin, 10

Printing: Ten Brink, Meppel, The Netherlands
Binding: Stürtz, Würzburg, Germany